HEALTHY EATING

Recipes for the Asian Palate

Chef **Nicholas Pillai**   Dietitian **Indra Balaratnam**

TIMES EDITIONS

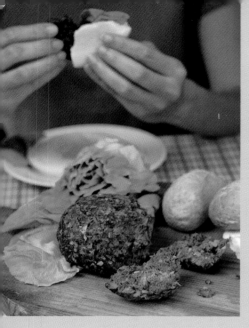

Chef
Nicholas Pillai

Managing Editor
Jamilah Mohd Hassan

Editor
Selina Kuo

Art Direction/Designer
Lynn Chin Nyuk Ling

Photographer
Suan I. Lim

Props Sourcing
Joycelyn George

Production Co-ordinator
Nor Sidah Haron

The publisher wishes to thank
Remix Home Shoppe Sdn Bhd
and
Royel Department Store
for the loan and use of their tableware.

© 2004 Marshall Cavendish International (Asia) Private Limited
Published by Times Editions – Marshall Cavendish
An imprint of Marshall Cavendish International (Asia) Private Limited
A member of Times Publishing Limited
Times Centre, 1 New Industrial Road, Singapore 536196
Tel: (65) 6213 9288   Fax: (65) 6285 4871
E-mail: te@sg.marshallcavendish.com
Online Bookstore: http://www.timesone.com.sg/te

Malaysian Office:
Federal Publications Sdn Berhad (General & Reference Publishing) (3024-D)
Times Subang, Lot 46, Persiaran Teknologi Subang
Subang Hi-Tech Industrial Park
Batu Tiga, 40000 Shah Alam
Selangor Darul Ehsan, Malaysia
Tel: (603) 5635 2191   Fax: (603) 5635 2706
E-mail: cchong@tpg.com.my

National Library Board (Singapore) Cataloguing in Publication Data

Pillai, Nicholas.
Healthy eating : recipes for the Asian palate / chef, Nicholas Pillai ; dietitian, Indra Balaratnam. —
Singapore : Times Editions, 2004.
p. cm.
ISBN : 981-232-709-6

1. Cookery, Asian. I. Balaratnam, Indra. II. Title

TX724.5.A1
641.595 — dc21   SLS2004023984

Printed in Singapore by Times Graphics (Pte) Ltd

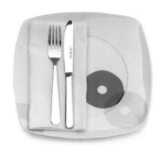

CONTENTS

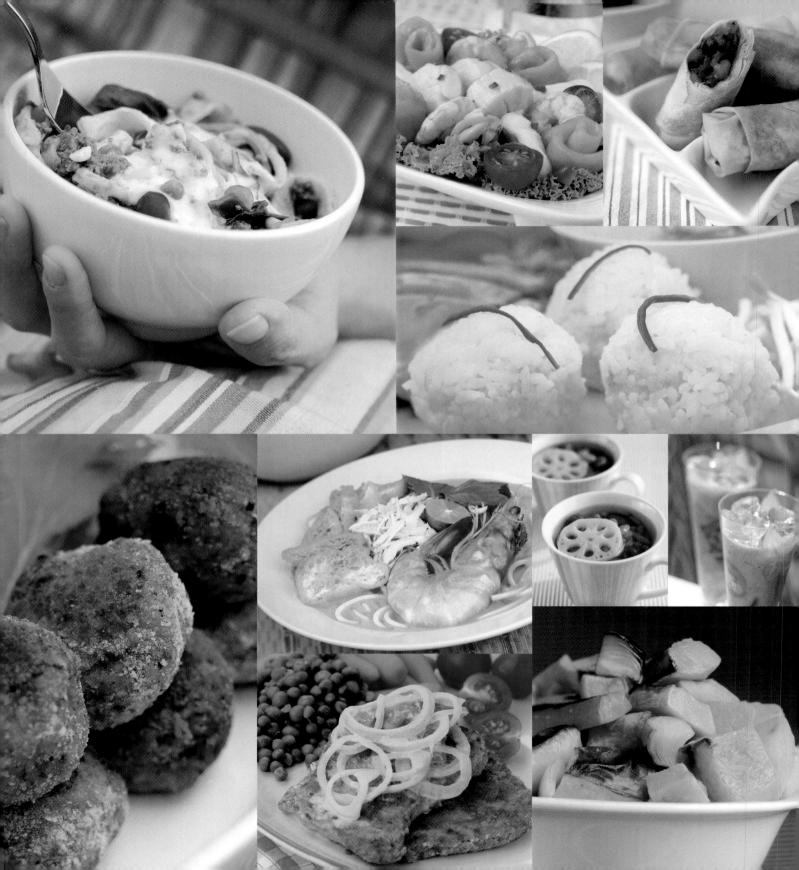

INTRODUCTION

Eating is a way of life. Some eat to live, but a majority live to eat. It's the 'foodie' in each of us that makes us that way. While food is the very melting pot in every culture, having a body that looks like a melting pot at the end of it all is certainly not very cultural!

In this day and age, people are constantly worried about cholesterol, fat and other dietary bad guys. There is no such thing as bad food, however, and in fact, food is the very essence that gives us energy and pep. Without it, we would be constantly hungry, grumpy and weak. Tell me, how can you be healthy when you're not happy? Hmm, maybe that's food for thought.

We could not agree more that food should be enjoyed and savoured wholeheartedly but it is difficult to enjoy your food when, at the back of your head, you're also worried about piling on the kilos. That's why this book represents the happy union of a 'foodie' and a dietitian — sharing our personal tips and know-how on making delicious, healthy meals. We have made eating healthy a lifestyle and have found it to be the best way to enjoy good food while watching our health. We've banished the word "diet" from our vocabulary!

This book contains a rich collection of Asian recipes cooked with good health in mind. What we've done is maintain the aromatic Asian ingredients and spices but resolved to cook them with less oil and fatty ingredients. The result is the dream of a 'foodie' — delicious food without massive dietary culprits.

Don't get us wrong, though, this is not a fat-free cookbook (who wants to eat cardboard?). The recipes here are good, old-fashioned Asian recipes that have been reinterpreted in a conscientious, healthy way. They are light but no less tasty, so you can enjoy these recipes in moderation without feeling the pangs of guilt that follow overdoing yourself with too much food.

We sincerely hope you will enjoy cooking and savouring these wholesome, Asian-inspired offerings.

From our kitchens to your heart,

Indra and Nicholas

GETTINGSTARTEDONHEALTHYEATING

Healthier eating starts with an intention. Does "I think I'm a blimp, where's my fairy godmother to slim me down?" sound familiar? While vanity is good motivation for a short-term goal, you're more likely to stick to healthier eating habits if you constantly remind yourself that you want to eat well to maintain good health. Diseases such as coronary heart disease, hypertension, Type 2 or adult-onset diabetes, gout, and even certain cancers can follow from one's overall diet and lifestyle. To fight the statistics and put the odds in your favour, change your mind set. Don't just do it for vanity, think body, mind and soul!

The Food Guide Pyramid — A Road Map To Healthy Eating

Healthy eating is all about choices. The adage "You are what you eat" has some truth. The good news is that there is no such thing as good or bad foods. All foods provide you with some nutrients that are important for your health. There's only good and bad NUTRITION. So, learn here how to create for yourself a lifelong eating plan worthy of nourishing your body, mind and soul.

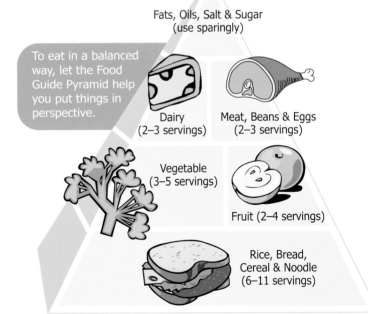

Fats, Oils, Salt & Sugar
(use sparingly)

To eat in a balanced way, let the Food Guide Pyramid help you put things in perspective.

Dairy
(2–3 servings)

Meat, Beans & Eggs
(2–3 servings)

Vegetable
(3–5 servings)

Fruit (2–4 servings)

Rice, Bread,
Cereal & Noodle
(6–11 servings)

Some important reminders about the pyramid

- Infants and children below the age of 12 should not follow the pyramid. Their dietary needs are different. Consult a paediatrician and a qualified dietitian for help on children's nutrition.

- All five basic food groups contribute different nutrients important to your diet, so make sure you eat foods from each group to avoid deficiencies in essential vitamins and minerals.

- Variety is key — don't get stuck in a diet rut! Select different types of food from each food group as much and as often as possible.

- Be conscious of how your food is cooked. Foods that are boiled, steamed, lightly pan-fried, grilled or baked are better choices.

A GUIDE TO DEFINING "ONE SERVING" FOR THE FOOD GROUPS

RICE, BREAD, CEREAL & NOODLE GROUP

Recommended daily servings: 6 to 11

Major nutrients: Starch, Fibre, B vitamins, Iron, Magnesium, Folic acid and Zinc

- 1 slice of bread
- ½ a hotdog or hamburger bun
- 4 small crackers
- 1 medium muffin
- 1 cup of breakfast cereal
- ½ cup of oats
- ½ cup of rice
- 1 cup of rice porridge
- 1 medium potato or other tubers

MEAT, BEANS & EGGS GROUP

Recommended daily servings: 2 to 3

Major nutrients: Protein, Niacin, Iron, Vitamin B6, Zinc, Thiamin and Vitamin B12 (in animal choices only)

- 100 g of cooked lean meat, fish or poultry (about the size of a deck of cards)
- 2 eggs
- 180 g of tofu
- 1 cup of cooked dried beans or peas (legumes)
- 4 Tbsp of peanut butter
- ½ cup of nuts or seeds

FRUIT GROUP

Recommended daily servings: 2 to 4

Major nutrients: Vitamin C, Fibre and Vitamin A

- 1 whole medium fruit (1 cup chopped)
- ¼ cup dried fruit
- ½ cup of canned fruit
- ¾ cup of fresh fruit juice

VEGETABLE GROUP

Recommended daily servings: 3 to 5

Major nutrients: Vitamin A, Vitamin C, Folic Acid, Magnesium and Fibre

- ½ cup of cooked vegetables
- 1 cup of raw vegetables
- ¾ cup of vegetable juice

DAIRY GROUP

Recommended daily servings: 2 to 3

Major nutrients: Calcium, Riboflavin, Protein, Potassium and Zinc

- 1 cup of milk or yoghurt
- 2 slices of cheese
- 2 cups of cottage cheese
- 1½ cups of ice cream or frozen yoghurt

HOW MUCH SHOULD YOU BE EATING DAILY?

If you are	An Average Woman / An Elderly Person	A Teenage Girl / An Active Woman / An Average Man	A Teenage Boy / An Active Man
You will need	1,600 calories per day	2,200 calories per day	2,800 calories per day
Rice, Bread, Cereal & Noodle group	6	9	11
Vegetable group	3	4	5
Fruit group	2	3	4
Meat, Beans & Eggs group	2	2	3
Dairy group	2	3	3

FATS

Fats have a bad reputation because obesity is problem that is affecting adults and children around the world. Even in Asia, we are not spared. We are at a stage where the stereotypically 'svelte' Asian is now commonly becoming overweight. Apart from sedentary lifestyles, health experts believe that eating too much fat is also a cause of people becoming overweight and developing health problems such as heart disease and Type 2 diabetes to name a couple.

Fat plays an amazing role in your body. It helps to transport vitamins A, D, E and K throughout the body, and it provides essential fatty acids that the body cannot make on its own. Plus, a certain level of fat is present in your body to cushion and protect major organs.

Fats are divided into three categories:

Saturated fat: Animal fat, coconut and palm oils, chicken skin, egg yolk, full cream dairy products.

Monounsaturated fat: Nuts, as well as olive and canola oils.

Polyunsaturated fat: Safflower, sunflower, corn, soybean and flaxseed oils. Also, Omega-3 fatty acids that are predominantly found in deep-sea fish such as mackerel, tuna and salmon.

From a health standpoint, eating foods high in saturated fat will put you at risk of coronary heart disease, higher cholesterol levels and obesity. Strive to replace saturated fat with monounsaturated and polyunsaturated alternatives. Just because the latter two are considered better for you, however, doesn't mean that you should be guzzling them down. An average adult who consumes 2,000 calories daily needs only about 65 grams of fat a day. Remember that a tablespoon of cooking oil has about 15 grams of fat, so about 4 tablespoons of cooking oil will be enough to meet your requirements for the day!

Simple Ways to Cut Down on Excess Fat

- Switch to low-fat (skimmed) dairy products such as milk, yogurt, cottage cheese, cream and cheese.

- Go easy on butter, spreads, salad dressings and cooking oil. Use spray oil, a nifty cooking invention.

- Choose the leanest cuts of meat or poultry you can find. Always trim off excess fat from meat and skin from poultry. If you want to make a moist roast, leave the skin and fat on, but use a baking tray with a grill on top of it so that the fat drippings can drain away. Then, remove the skin and excess fat before eating.

- Avoid store-bought mince because skin and fat are often ground along with the meat. Instead, buy lean meat or skinned chicken and mince at home using a food processor.

- Use good quality stainless steel or nonstick crockery. They may be more expensive but they allow you to minimise the use of oil in your cooking.

- Replace coconut cream, which is high in saturated fat, with a similarly creamy but far healthier substitute — unsweetened soy or rice milk.

CHOLESTEROL

Cholesterol makes up cell membranes, builds healthy nerves and is the founding block for healthy cells. It is an essential substance to our health but many of us eat more cholesterol than we need.
Our liver primarily manufactures enough cholesterol to meet the needs of our body. The cholesterol we get from food is supposed to complement what our body makes.

In simplified terms, just remember this — LDL (low density lipoproteins) are the BADDIES because they clog up your arteries over time. HDL (high density lipoproteins) are the GOODIES because they clear excess LDL and plaque from artery walls.

Only animal food products, e.g. meats, seafood, dairy, butter, animal oils and eggs, contain cholesterol. Plant foods, e.g. vegetables, beans, lentils, fruits, margarine and vegetable oils, have ZERO cholesterol.

Simple Ways to Cut Down on Cholesterol

- Eat moderate amounts of animal products. Use beans and lentils as complementary sources of protein.
- Limit your intake of foods high in saturated fat, e.g. fatty meats, desserts, snack foods and oils.
- Choose foods high in fibre, e.g. vegetables, fruit, beans and grains.
- Adopt a healthy lifestyle with moderate to high intensity exercises on a daily basis.

SALT

Gone are the days when salt was the food of the kings. It may have been so back then simply because they did not have as many ingredients as we have at our disposal today.

Throughout this book, you will notice that salt is kept to a minimum in the recipes and is often defined as "to taste". Health reasons aside, remember, especially when you are entertaining, to be careful with salt because once you over-salt something, it is almost irreparable. Salt can overpower almost every ingredient in your dish if you are not careful.

Simple Ways to Cut Down on Salt

- Taste your food first before adding any salt. Remember, too, that when food is hot, it seems less salty because the heat hits your tongue before the taste.
- Read food labels to check their sodium content.
- Go easy on processed sauces and seasonings, e.g. soy sauce, ketchup, MSG and other flavour enhancers. A little goes a long way.

FIBRE

Fibre-rich foods are high in nutrients and have a special health mechanism. Health experts rave that they can help to lower cholesterol levels, ease constipation and regulate blood sugar levels.

Fibre is divided into two categories:

Soluble fibre: Oatmeal, bran, legumes, fruits and vegetables.

Insoluble fibre: Wheat, bran, whole grains, stems of vegetables, cereals and fruits.

For all its goodness, the average person still doesn't eat enough fibre in a day. The recommended amount is between 20 and 30 grams a day.

Simple Ways to Enrich Your Fibre Intake

- Eat more foods that are high in fibre, e.g. vegetables, beans, legumes, seeds, nuts, grains and cereals, on a daily basis.
- Throw beans into dishes or use wholemeal flour in your baking.
- When eating out, always order a side of vegetables to complement a quick meal. For example, if you're having a bowl of *laksa* for lunch at a food court, order some vegetables from the mixed rice stall. Alternatively, have a generous salad with your chicken chop.
- Snack on a small serving of nuts and seeds rather than mindlessly munch on oily crisps. Steam up a batch of chickpeas or beans to eat with your rice or when you need something to munch on when watching the telly.
- Juicing fruits like an apple in a juicer is a nice treat, but it also removes the skin. It's always better to eat the fruit fresh, with the skin if possible.
- High-fibre breakfast cereals aren't only for breakfast. If you're totally unable to cook a meal, then a bowl of wholegrain cereal with milk is a fantastically complete substitute. Cereal without milk is also a great munching snack to replace cookies.

Nutrient Analysis Chart

This is how much an average healthy adult on a 2,000 calorie a day intake needs.

Nutrient	Average amount per day
Protein	0.75 g of protein per kg of your body weight
Carbohydrates	300 g
Total fat	Less than 65 g
Cholesterol	Less than 300 mg
Fibre	20–25 g
Sodium	Less than 2,400 mg

SPECIALPREPARATIONTECHNIQUES

Nicholas' Guide to Making Stock

To lead a healthy lifestyle, sometimes we have to do away with a few conveniences that we have picked up along the way. One convenience is using bouillons and stock cubes to enhance the flavour of our food. It is not only high in fat, but also horribly high in salt and flavour enhancers, all of which do little for your health. If you don't believe that stock cubes have a high fat content, try boiling one in water, then refrigerating the cooled liquid. Knowing full well that you did not add any oil to the water, you will still find a layer of oil hardened at the surface.

Stocks are the very essence of making tasty foods in this book. Through the years, I have found that a tasty stock will make your food much richer without having to add ingredients like milk, cream and coconut milk.

Stocks are not hard to prepare. You will have to be in the kitchen for the first 15 minutes to skim off the scum but after that, you can carry on with your work while it sits on the stove. I have recommended three hours for the two meat stocks (refer to p.12), but you can cook it for a little shorter if you like. The longer the cooking time, the better it will taste though, that's for sure.

Remember to cool it and store it as soon as possible because there is no seasoning or flavouring in your stock. This means that it will go bad rather quickly. Even cooler climates are not exempt, so please be mindful of storing your stock. It will otherwise be such a waste of effort if the stock turns rancid before it is used. That has happened to me once, and I was rather displeased. Actually, I was rather angry because my flatmate forgot to put it in the freezer. Four hours of simmering and it all went to waste the next morning. A piece of advice — prepare your stocks early in the day so you can store it away early too.

Another thing different about my stocks is that I do not use a bouquet garni, a combination of flavour-enhancing herbs and spices. I feel that there is no need to because in Asian cooking, the stock is used as part of already flavourful dishes and the combination could confuse and spoil the end product. However, if you feel you prefer a stock with more kick, feel free to add whatever you like to it. Remember that these recipes reflect only what I like. When you start using these recipes, tweak them and make them yours.

Basic Chicken Stock

Chicken bones	500 g, cleaned and washed
Hot water	4–5 litres
Onion	1/2
Garlic	1 clove

- Combine bones and water in a pot. Bring to the boil and sustain for a few minutes. Skim off scum from the surface.
- Reduce heat. Add onion and garlic. Simmer for about 3 hours or until liquid is halved. Remove from heat and leave to cool.
- Put cooled stock in freezer for a few hours so fat will separate.
- Remove stock from freezer and discard solidified fat collected at the surface. Strain before storing.

Basic Beef Stock

Beef bones	500 g, cleaned and washed
Onion	1
Garlic	1–2 cloves
Black peppercorns	5–6
Hot water	3–5 litres or more

- Boil water over high heat. Add bones and leave to boil for a few minutes. Skim off blood and scum from the surface.
- Reduce heat. Add onion and garlic. Simmer for 3 hours or until liquid is halved. Remove from heat and leave to cool.
- Put cooled stock in freezer for a few hours so fat will separate.
- Remove soup from freezer and discard fat collected at the surface. Strain before storing.

Basic Fish or Seafood Stock

Fish bones or prawn (shrimp) shells	250 g or more
Hot water	1 litre

- Combine fish bones or prawn shells and water in a pot. Boil for about 20 minutes. Remove from heat and leave to cool.
- Strain before storing.

Basic Vegetable Stock

Onion	1, large, peeled and roughly chopped
Garlic	2, peeled and roughly chopped
Celery	500 g, roughly chopped
Carrot	1, roughly chopped
Cabbage leaves	5–6
Parsley	1 sprig
White peppercorns	3–4
Black peppercorns	5–6
Dried bay leaves	2–3
Water	5 litres

- Wash all the vegetables properly.
- Bring water to the boil over high heat. Add vegetables and bring to another boil.
- Reduce heat and simmer for 3–4 hours.
- Strain and store in freezer for later use.

Skimming Off Fat

Don't waste your time spooning out the fat from the surface of your stock or soup! Don't waste your time with all those gadgets you find in the supermarkets! Don't waste your time placing it in the refrigerator either, because it is generally not cold enough.

Instead, freeze the stock or soup for at least one hour so that the fat it contains will separate and solidify at the top. Sometimes you will be so surprised to see the thickness of the fat accumulated. Throw it away.

Now, you have almost fat-free soup. I say almost because we have a tendency to add a whole lot of fatty ingredients and not bother to skim off the fat once more. If you add meat or chicken, redo the whole process. Always put in the soft vegetables last.

Storing Stocks

I store my meat and chicken stocks in the freezer for many, many months. As long as you do not keep taking it out and putting it back, it should be good for a long while. I never make fish stock or prawn stock unless desperate. It is my opinion that fish stock should only be used when cooking with seafood. I never use fish stock to cook meats because I do not like the taste. The decision is yours, however. You may like the taste or you may know people who do.

One more point. Once you become a habitual maker of stocks, label and date them. Dating containers of stock reminds you to use the older ones first. You should also label and clearly identify the different stocks you have. I have learnt to do this because my brother-in-law Matt is allergic to all things poultry and I have to be extra careful with the ingredients, including those that went into making the stock.

- **Iced stock cubes**

  When you have cooked a very rich stock, you can transfer a quantity to ice cube trays to freeze. Not all dishes require large amounts of stock, so it is handy to have small quantities in the form of ice cubes. One or two cubes is enough to give your stir-fry dishes or just about anything you are cooking some added flavour. Never return defrosted stock to the freezer. Thawing stock is a breeding ground for bacteria.

- **Store bowlfuls in plastic bags or containers**

  Store prepared stocks in plastic bags or containers that hold enough for the preparation of one meal for yourself, for two or however many in the household. You can also store stock in ziploc bags, which allows you to lay them flat and pile them up in the freezer.

- **Storing fish stock**

  As a rule, I do not freeze fish stock to keep as it does not take very long to make. Anyhow the process of cleanly storing prawn shells or fish bones in the freezer is rather tedious and not worth the trouble for stock in my opinion. When you need fish stock for a seafood dish, just use the skin or parts of the seafood you have already purchased for the dish to make the stock fresh.

Toasting Spices, Nuts or Seeds

Spread out the desired spices, nuts or seeds in a nonstick pan. Toast over low heat for 5 to 10 minutes, stirring constantly. Alternatively, spread them out on a baking tray and bake for about 10 minutes in a 180°C (350°F) oven.

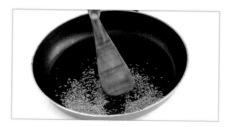

Removing Fat from Meat

Trim off all visible traces of fat from meats. Remove the skin of poultry. Sometimes, it's not easy to remove as much fat from raw meats as you would like. Lamb is one fine example. In such instances, it is easier to remove the remaining fat after the meat is cooked. That way, the little fat or skin left on the meat helps it to stay tender and moist while being baked or grilled. Every cook's nightmare is for meats to be hard and dry like a brick.

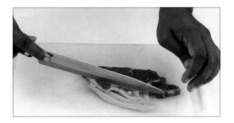

Using Fresh Herbs

A fuss-free way to cut fresh herbs is to put them in a cup and snip them with kitchen scissors. If you are unable to obtain a herb fresh, use the dried variety. When substituting, the quantity to be added is one-third the amount for the herb fresh, i.e. 10 g dried = 30 g fresh.

Separating Eggs

Over a bowl, crack an egg such that the shell is split into halves. Carefully move the egg yolk back and forth, from one half to the other, while you allow the egg white to fall into the bowl below. Alternatively, buy an egg separator, which you can find in household shops.

Searing Onions and Garlic

You will find that almost every other recipe is telling you to sear onions and garlic, sometimes just before squirting the spray oil and at other times with a little water or stock to bring out the flavour and to prevent burning.

If the onions are roughly chopped, then throw them directly into a hot pan to sear. Searing means actually hearing the onions go *searrrrrrrrrr*! Add in a little water and you will see the brownness of the onion pieces emerge and this makes them more aromatic. You may also spray a little oil at this moment.

When the ingredients are minced, however, spray the oil before adding in the finely cut ingredients. Once the searing sound begins, add a little stock or water to carry on the cooking of the ingredients and the infusing of their flavours.

Herbs and Spices

Herbs and spices bring out the goodness of any food. Do not go overboard with it, of course, but make it a point to use it more often than salt when it comes to flavouring your foods. Sometimes, you have to take chances with these herbs and spices. After all, a lot of our cooking experiences are the fruits of experimenting, so why don't you give it a try too and unleash your spice creativity. Spices are best kept in the refrigerator if you are going to take a long time to finish them, which is often the case.

Soy Milk and Rice Milk

Indra and I used soy and rice milk for recipes in this book because we found them to be a nice change from skimmed milk. They not only bring about a creamier, richer texture to the gravy, but also are great alternatives for people who are lactose intolerant.

One thing to note, though, is that only unsweetened soy and rice milk should be used. In many parts of Asia, soy milk drinks are available in cans, bottles and cartons, but these have a lot of sugar in them and are not what we use for the recipes. Unsweetened soy milk is really thick and creamy, just like full cream milk.

Using Spray Oil

Spray oils can be found in just about all supermarkets. While it is a little more expensive, you will find that it lasts longer than your usual bottle or tin of oil. The reason for this is because you spray on the precise amount you need. One spray should safely fry you an egg and even your bacon slices for breakfast. Always use low heat with spray oil as it tends to burn rather quickly due to the small quantity used. In some instances, you need to throw in the ingredients as soon as you spray your pan to prevent the oil from smoking. Generally, to coat a cooking surface, spray from 10 cm or more away (*top*). Hold spray oil closer to cover a smaller but more concentrated area (*bottom*).

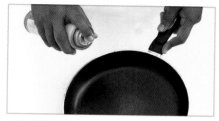
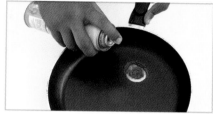

TRICKS OF THE TRADE TO A FASTER MEAL

- Even if you think you can't cook an egg, cooking is something you can learn to love. Many a time, we hear people grumble when they look at a recipe. "It's too long!" "It looks so difficult!" These are all excuses because like anything else we do in our life, all it needs is a little planning.

- Always have some minced ingredients on hand. Mince a little bit more of each ingredient, e.g. garlic or ginger, every time you cook and store in it in the refrigerator. These ingredients keep well for a few days in the refrigerator if they are stored in airtight containers. It is also a good idea to invest in a few small containers to store these ingredients.

- There are some ingredients that are more difficult to handle than others. Galangal, for example, is a lot harder than many other ingredients to even blend (process). Once you have embarked on the task, it pays for you to process such ingredients in bulk and then freeze for future use. Furthermore, if you get your hands on young galangal, grab the lot, I tell you! It is so difficult to find young galangal most times.

- As for meats, be nice to your butcher and he will cut the meat the way you like it. Marinate the meat in advance. In fact, the longer it marinates, the faster it will cook. This not only cuts down waiting time, but also improves the taste.

- It is a good idea to invest in a good quality food processor as you can use it in a myriad of ways, from mincing meat and fish to slicing onions and mincing garlic, all in a few seconds.

- A liquidizer is also a must for making those nice shakes and juices. Try not to use the same jug for other foods as odours may linger and your delicious strawberry milk shake may bear hints of lemon grass.

- A good microwave oven is something a modern, busy person cannot live without. Do not make a habit out of cooking in it, but use it for reheating. It is especially useful when reheating soups because it heats to just the right temperature without destroying the vegetables. Sometimes, leftovers look much better reheated in the microwave oven than they would have over stove top heat.

Nicholas

I started to really appreciate nice soups when I lived overseas. I guess cold winter nights had something to do with it. Also, exams tended to be during winter and soups were the fastest meals to make. You see, my friends and I would have messed around in class all semester and timesaving became important so that we could study for dear life. Soups were 'in' during those periods.

Soups are ideal for those who work late and choose to eat late at night. Because eating heavy meals late in the day is a no-no, try a warm, nutritious soup instead. It will help you go to bed feeling rather satisfied and not gluggy.

Make your soups a day or even a few days ahead, perhaps on the weekends. Add in the fresh vegetables only on the day it is to be served, however. Start with the strong-flavoured ingredients like onions, herbs and, of course, the meat of your choice. Refrigerating or freezing the soup also enables you to remove the fat that solidifies at the surface before consuming it.

Indra

I never truly appreciated soups until I stayed in the US for several years and experienced cold weather. I'm telling you, when the chills hit your bones, there's nothing more satisfying than a steaming bowl of soup. It's no wonder that when people are down with the flu, soup is the first thing they think of to help clear the sinuses.

Nowadays, you can buy canned and powdered soups from your supermarkets but these ready-made soups are unfortunately very high in sodium and flavour enhancers. A diet too high in sodium can cause water retention and is not advisable for those with certain diseases such as kidney failure or hypertension.

Believe it or not, soups are actually one of the easiest things to make. You literally boil all the ingredients together in a large pot and while that is happening, you can take a shower or do a crossword puzzle. The 'hardest' part is cutting up all the ingredients but I'm sure you can get around that!

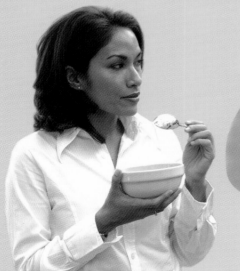

SOUPS

LENTILSOUP

Nick's culinary jottings: I find this soup to be rather filling and satisfying and it covers all the food groups needed for a wholesome day. Based on my own experience, I don't think kids would really like this soup. Frankly, I hated lentils most of my life and only started eating them after tasting all the different varieties when I lived overseas. For some reason, only a few types of lentils were available in Malaysia, until now that is. I sometimes use this thick soup as a meal replacement.

Preparation time : 20 minutes
Cooking time : 40–45 minutes
Serves 4

Ingredients

Water	500 ml
Cloves	5–6
Star anise	2
Cinnamon stick	1
Cardamoms	2
Stock	1 litre
Orange lentils	55 g
Green lentils	55 g
Mung dhal	55 g
Carrot	1, thickly sliced
Onion	1, peeled and cubed
Garlic	2 cloves, peeled and minced
Potatoes	2, cut into large cubes and parboiled
Salt and pepper	to taste
Dry-fried fennel	2 tsp or 1 fresh stalk
Black pepper	to taste (optional)

Method

- Bring water to the boil. Add cloves, star anise, cinnamon and cardamoms. Leave to boil until liquid is halved.

- Add stock, then lentils, dhal and carrot at the same time. Bring to another boil.

- Simmer for a few minutes, then add onion and garlic. Simmer a while more.

- Add potatoes. Leave to simmer for 10 minutes. Add salt and pepper to taste.

- Do not over-boil. Soup should be slightly clear and not too murky. You should be able to see the differently coloured lentils.

- Serve with fennel and freshly cracked black pepper if used.

Note: **Mung dhal refers to mung (green) beans that have been skinned and split.**

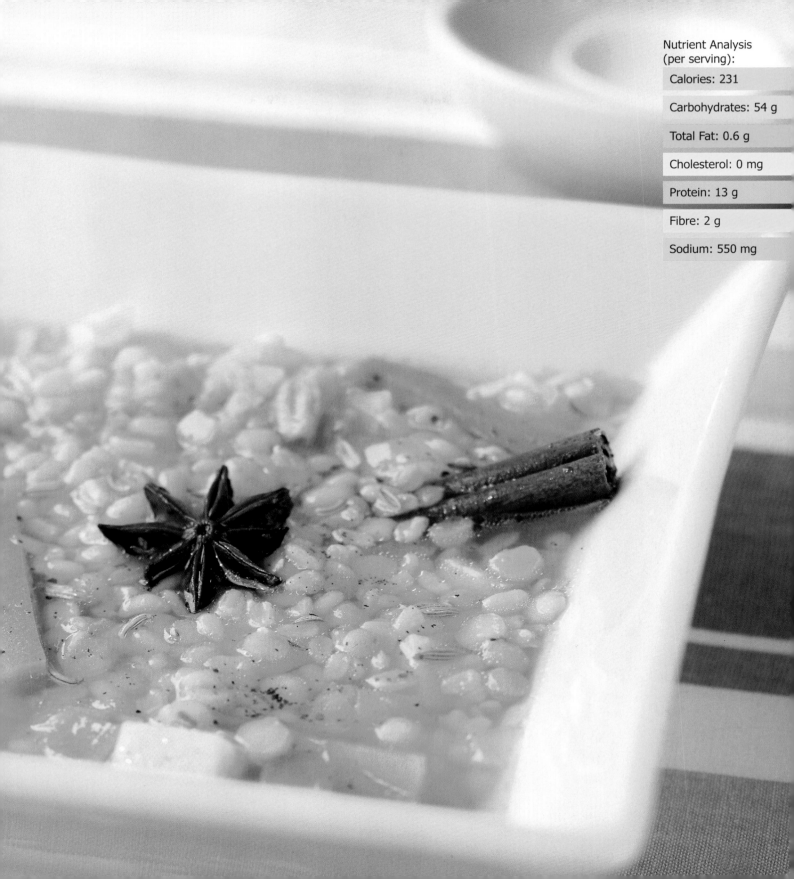

Nutrient Analysis
(per serving):

Calories: 279

Carbohydrates: 40 g

Total fat: 3 g

Cholesterol: 0 mg

Protein: 14 g

Fibre: 5 g

Sodium: 120 mg

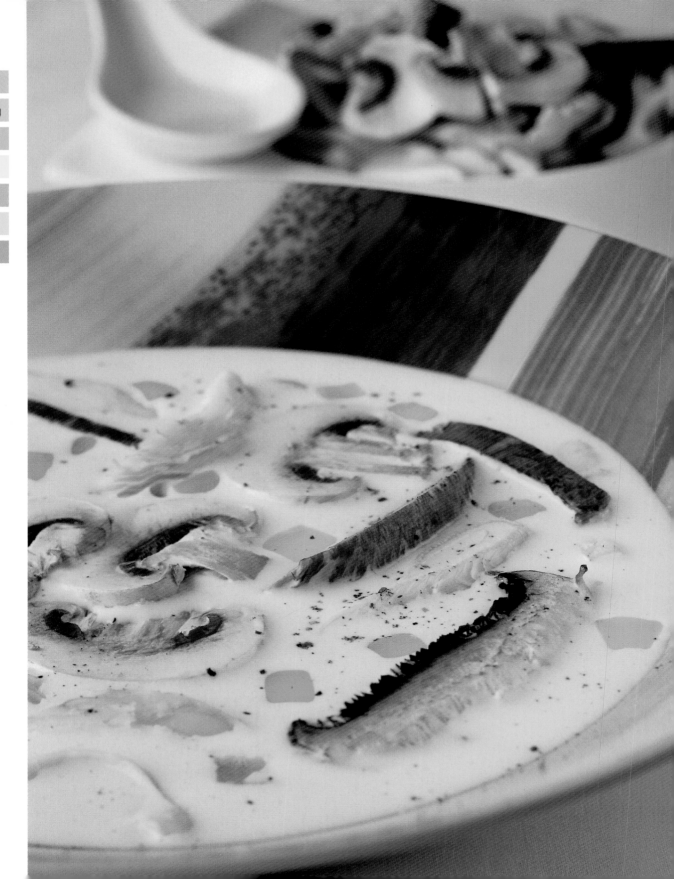

CREAM OF MUSHROOM SOUP

Nick's culinary jottings: Use fresh mushrooms for heaven's sake. In Asia, we are blessed with just as many types of mushrooms as there are in the West. Any mushroom can be used for this recipe. Just make sure you don't get all the dark-coloured ones or you will end up with black and creamy mushroom soup.

Preparation time : 10 minutes
Cooking time : 40–45 minutes
Serves 4

Method

- Slice half the shiitake mushrooms. Reserve slices for garnishing. Also reserve half the button mushroom slices for garnishing. Keep garnish under cling film (plastic wrap) to prevent discolouring.

- In a pot, sear onion until lightly brown. A mild brown is good enough or it is likely to burn. Add a little water at a time as you do this. It should take around 5 minutes and ensures that flavours infuse the liquid.

- Add oyster and shiitake mushrooms. Lightly brown them as well. Then, add flour and whisk to prevent lumps. When done, add stock and bring to the boil.

- Add remaining mushrooms. Simmer for about 10 minutes. Soup should not be boiling but gently simmering. If soup is too thick, add more stock or some soy milk.

- Add salt and pepper to taste. Simmer for 5 minutes. Remove from heat and leave to cool. Alternatively, add soy milk after salt and pepper, then simmer 10 minutes more for a chunky mushroom soup.

- For smooth soup, blend (process) cooled liquid to desired consistency, then return to pot and bring to the boil. Add soy milk and simmer a while. Serve garnished with mushroom slices.

Ingredients

Fresh shiitake mushrooms	100 g
Button mushrooms	100 g, sliced
Onion	1, large, peeled and chopped
Water	250 ml
Oyster mushrooms	200 g, roughly chopped
Plain (all-purpose) flour	60 g
Stock	500 ml
Dried Chinese mushrooms	50 g, soaked, stems discarded, then boiled and roughly chopped
Salt and black pepper	to taste
Unsweetened soy milk	500 ml

TOMATO SOUP

Nick's culinary jottings: I drink this soup on days when I am feeling really gluggy or after I have feasted on a lot of rich foods the day before or just earlier in the day. Its light and tangy flavour is fresh and does not drown the senses. I have kept this soup properly covered in the refrigerator for five or six days and it still tasted excellent.

Preparation time : 10 minutes
Cooking time : 40–45 minutes
Serves 4

Ingredients

Red tomatoes	1 kg, quartered
Vegetable stock	1 litre
Garlic	3 cloves, peeled and minced
Bay leaves	2
Lemon grass (*serai*)	1 stalk, bruised
Black peppercorns	5–6
French beans	125 g, thinly sliced
Salt	to taste

Method

- Reserve a handful of quartered tomatoes. Finely chop the rest.
- Bring stock to the boil. Add finely chopped tomatoes, garlic, bay leaves, lemon grass and peppercorns. Simmer for about 30 minutes.
- Add remaining tomatoes and beans, then salt to taste. Simmer for 5 minutes more.
- Serve hot with bread. Personally, I love eating the soup with crackers broken on top.

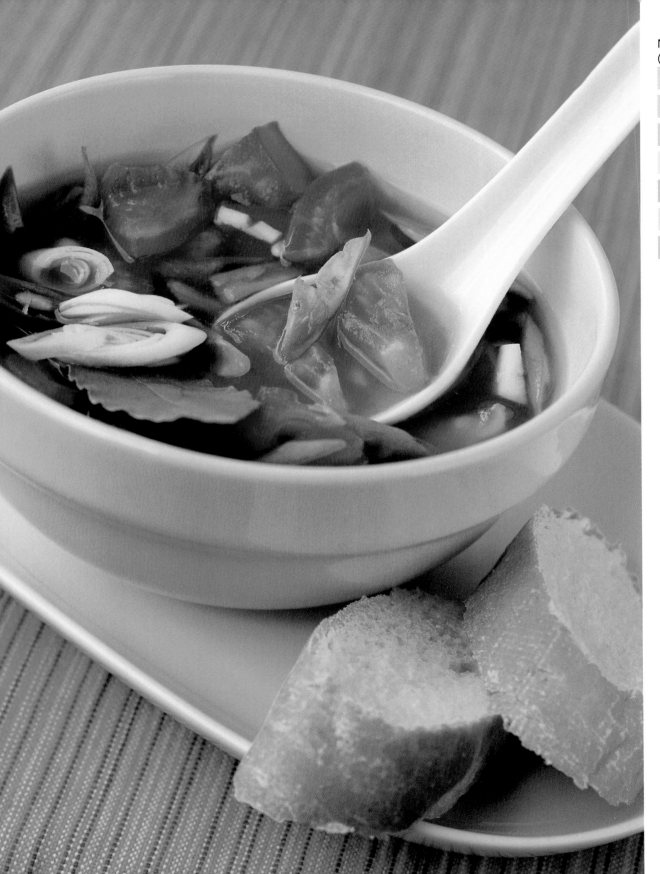

Nutrient Analysis
(per serving):

Calories: 69

Carbohydrates: 12 g

Total Fat: 0.5 g

Cholesterol: 0 mg

Protein: 4 g

Fibre: 2 g

Sodium: 575 mg

Nutrient Analysis
(per serving):

Calories: 253

Carbohydrates: 21 g

Total Fat: 9 g

Cholesterol: 73 mg

Protein: 22 g

Fibre: 3 g

Sodium: 640 mg

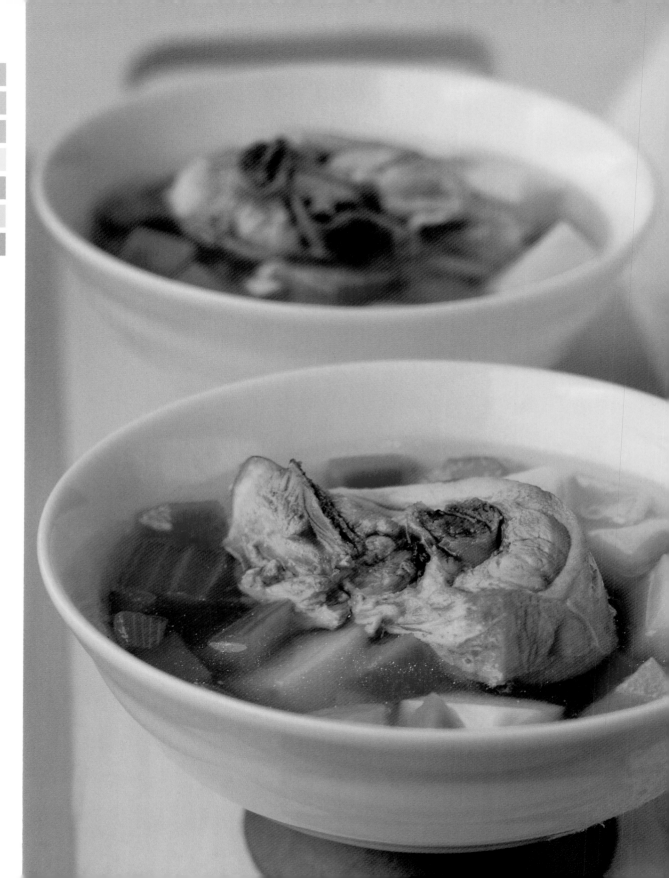

MAMA'S STYLE CHICKEN SOUP

Nick's culinary jottings: I've long wondered why a simple chicken soup often conjures up the mental image of a nice family lunch on a Sunday afternoon. I came to realise that it's possibly because it brings the best out of anyone. It changes the mood of the occasion, if not the whole atmosphere. This healthy recipe is so good and so economical too.

Preparation time : 15 minutes
Cooking time : 60 minutes
Serves 4

Method

- Combine chicken, stock, onions and garlic in a pot. Bring to the boil. Simmer for about 20 minutes. Remove from heat and leave to cool.

- Freeze cooled liquid for about 30 minutes or until fat solidifies on top. Discard fat. Remove and refrigerate chicken.

- Bring soup to the boil. Add celery and carrot. Boil for a few minutes, then add potatoes. Leave to simmer for 10 minutes. Add sugar, as well as salt and pepper to taste.

- Add coriander and leave to boil for a few minutes more.

- Return chicken to pot. Serve just like a broth. Easy to eat and no mess at the table. Remove garlic if you wish.

Ingredients

Chicken thighs	6, skinned and excess fat removed
Stock	1 litre
Onions	2, large, peeled and roughly chopped
Garlic	3–4 cloves, left whole
Celery	3 sticks, cubed
Carrot	1, large, peeled and cubed
Potatoes	2, large, peeled and cubed
Sugar	1 pinch
Salt and pepper	to taste
Coriander (cilantro) leaves	1 handful, roughly chopped

CHICKEN AND MANGO DUMPLINGS IN CLEAR BROTH

Nick's culinary jottings: I have a mango tree that fruits all year round for some reason, which leaves me with an abundance of the fruit a lot of the time. I quite by accident cooked this up one day and the result was rather pleasing. A simple stock can be used as the clear broth, or perhaps even the tomato soup before. Of course, then, it won't be clear but certainly different-tasting.

Preparation time : 30 minutes
Cooking time : 20 minutes
Serves 4

Ingredients

Minced chicken	250 g
Unripe mango	1, small, peeled and minced
Yam bean (*bang kuang*)	1, small, peeled and minced
Light soy sauce	1 tsp
Sugar	¼ tsp
Salt and pepper	to taste
Wonton skins	20
Egg white	1, lightly beaten
Onion	1, large, peeled and finely chopped
Chicken stock	1.5 litres

Garnishing

Julienned red capsicum (sweet bell pepper)

Julienned spring onions (scallions)

Julienned carrot

Method

- To make filling, combine chicken, mango, yam bean, soy sauce and sugar. Add salt and pepper to taste. Mix well. Set aside for 10 minutes.

- To make a dumpling, take a square wonton skin and turn it 45 degrees so that it is a diamond looking on. Spoon some filling onto half the diamond. Fold other half over filling and seal edges with egg white. Repeat until skins are used up.

- Sauté onion with a little stock until fragrant, not brown. Add remaining stock and bring to the boil.

- Add dumplings and simmer until cooked. Drain dumplings and transfer into serving bowls.

- Adjust broth to taste with more salt and pepper if desired. Ladle over dumplings.

- Garnish before serving.

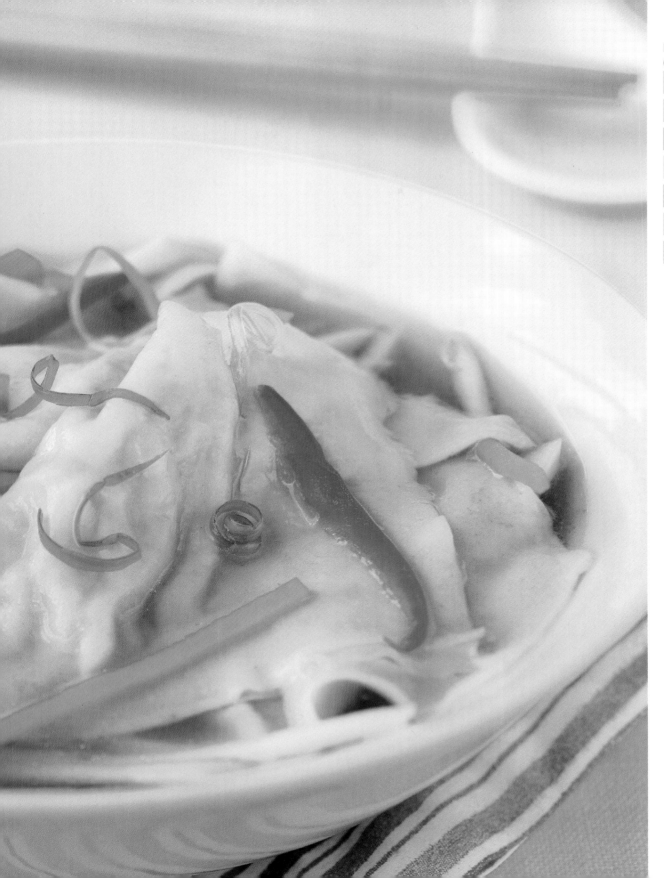

Nutrient Analysis
(per serving):

Calories: 136

Carbohydrates: 10 g

Total Fat: 5 g

Cholesterol: 55 mg

Protein: 13 g

Fibre: 1 g

Sodium: 380 mg

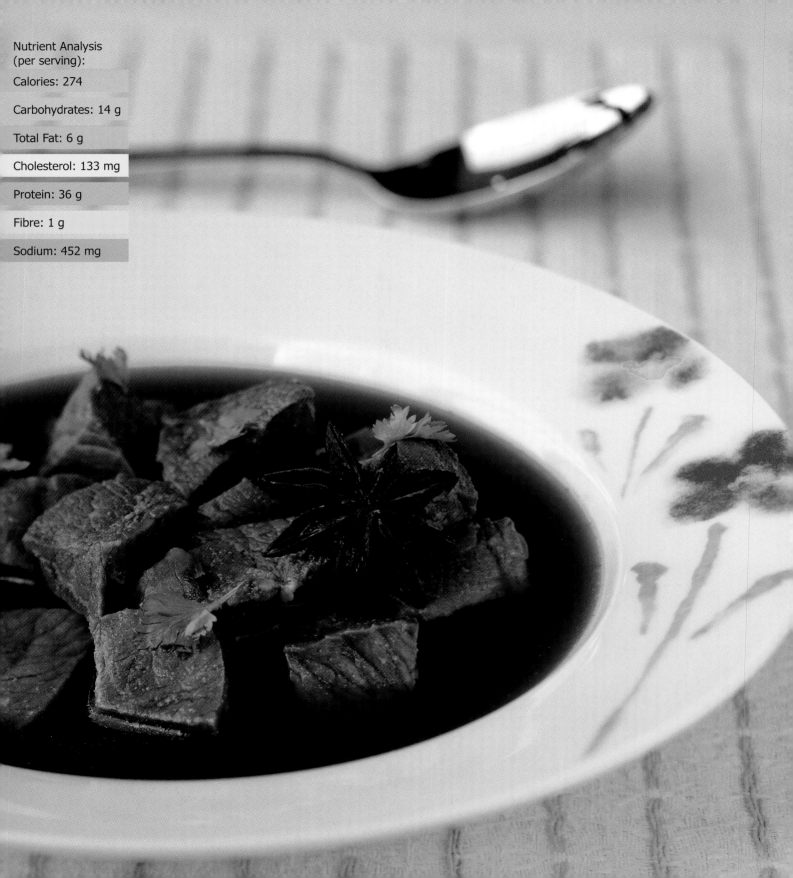

Nutrient Analysis
(per serving):

Calories: 274

Carbohydrates: 14 g

Total Fat: 6 g

Cholesterol: 133 mg

Protein: 36 g

Fibre: 1 g

Sodium: 452 mg

MUTTONSOUP(SUPKAMBING)

Nick's culinary jottings: I was never a fan of *sup kambing* simply because I always found it too oily. To me, such a glorious soup with ladles of oil overpowering everything is an absolute sore point. Although is it similar to oxtail soup, another fat piler so to speak, the rich assortment of spices here is simply a thrill to the palate. Try this easy-to-make yet healthy alternative. In place of coconut milk, I have used rice milk, which can be found in the larger supermarkets. I also love eating this with *ketupat* (compressed rice).

Preparation time : 20 minutes
Cooking time : 90 minutes
(excludes fat removal)
Serves 6

Method

- Blend (process) onions, garlic, galangal, ginger and green chillies together.

- Marinate meat with blended ingredients and roughly pounded spices combined, preferably overnight. Add a pinch of salt and pepper.

- Combine marinated meat, cardamoms, cloves, cinnamon and stock in a large pot. Bring to the boil. Simmer for about 1 hour. Remove from heat.

- Cool off in freezer and skim off fat. Don't be surprised to see the amount of fat floating.

- Return to the boil. Simmer until meat is tender. You may need more stock. Add salt and pepper to taste, then rice milk. Simmer for about 20 minutes more.

- Garnish with coriander. Serve hot.

Ingredients

Onions	3, large, peeled
Garlic	5 cloves, peeled
Galangal (*lengkuas*)	50 g
Ginger	50 g
Green chillies	3
Mutton or lamb chops	1 kg, excess fat removed
Fennel	2 tsp, roughly pounded
White poppy seeds	1 tsp, roughly pounded
Black peppercorns	2 Tbsp, roughly pounded
Coriander (cilantro) seeds	2 Tbsp, roughly pounded
Black cardamoms	5, lightly crushed
Cloves	4–5
Cinnamon sticks	2
Stock	2 litres
Salt and pepper	to taste
Rice milk	250 ml
Coriander (cilantro) leaves	

Nicholas

Ahhh! This is my second-favourite course of a meal, after dessert of course. I have always had this obsession with tiny morsels of foods for some reason. In fact, I used to fantasise about having platefuls of appetisers around the house so that I could pick at them whenever I pleased all day long.

Appetisers are crowd pleasers. They get everyone in the mood and a good start means a good meal all through. Most times, though, appetisers that please the eye, no matter how strange they may taste, can satisfy even discerning palates. I always start my parties with appetisers, but there are also people who fill themselves up with these finger foods and then ruin the rest of the meal. You know what they say, be a little mean and keep them keen.

Indra

The main problem with appetiser foods is that they are usually deep-fried, which is a sure-fire way to add on the fat grams to even the healthiest of food choices. Just think of your favourite pub grub snack foods — fried chicken wings, fried anchovies, fried spring rolls, chips or French fries. I rest my case! Also because they're small in size, you'd tend to wolf down way too many pieces before you feel full. All that and you haven't even reached your main course yet, *dahling*!

As Nicholas has so eloquently put it, appetiser foods are crowd pleasers. Basically, it gives people a chance to nibble on something while they mingle. What a lot of people don't realise is that healthier appetiser foods can be made by using other methods of cooking, i.e. baking, grilling, steaming, etc. Appetiser foods don't necessarily need to be fried. Change your mind set and your guests will thank you for being such a thoughtful, health-conscious host.

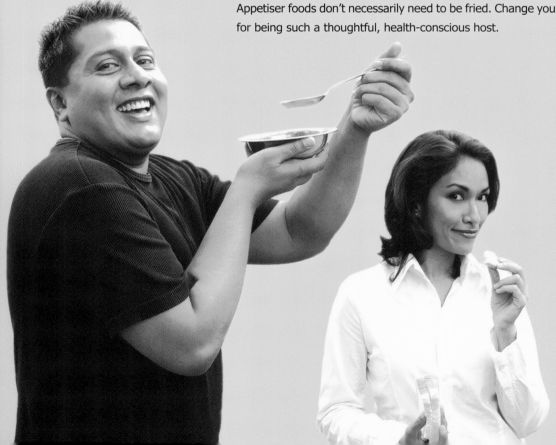

APPETISERS

SPRINGROLLS

Nick's culinary jottings: For some odd reason, spring rolls are a favourite the world over. Be it in Metropolitan New York or on the islands of Fiji, they are always on an Asian menu. There is no right or wrong recipe anymore because springs rolls have evolved over the years and in different cultures. Try this baked version. It is not so messy and more importantly, low in fat and healthy.

Preparation time : 30 minutes (includes wrapping of spring rolls)
Cooking time : 30 minutes (includes baking of spring rolls)
Serves 5

Ingredients

Spray oil	2 squirts
Garlic	2 cloves, peeled and minced
Stock	125 ml
Minced chicken	150 g
Dried Chinese mushrooms	3, soaked, boiled and thinly sliced
Salt	to taste
Ground black pepper	1 tsp
Sugar	1/2 tsp
Carrot	1, julienned
Purple cabbage leaves	6, spines removed and julienned
Coriander (cilantro) leaves	30 g
Spring roll skins (large)	20
Egg white	1, lightly beaten

Method

- Apply spray oil onto a saucepan. Sauté garlic. Add a little stock to prevent burning.

- Add chicken and fry until lightly cooked. Add mushrooms, then remaining stock. Season to taste with salt, pepper and sugar. Leave to simmer for about 5 minutes.

- Add carrot and cabbage. Stir thoroughly. Add coriander and stir well to mix. Remove from heat and leave to cool thoroughly. Do not overcook or vegetables will lose crunch.

- If there is excess liquid, drain vegetables using a colander. Reserve and freeze liquid to use as stock in future.

- To make a spring roll, take a piece of skin and turn it 45 degrees so that it is a diamond looking on. Arrange a length of filling just under widest part of diamond. Take bottom corner and fold toward centre over filling. Fold in both left and right corners, then roll up to top corner. Seal with egg white. Repeat until skins are used up.

- Preheat oven to 200°C (400°F). Heat baking tray for 10 minutes or until hot.

- Remove tray from oven and apply spray oil. Arrange spring rolls on tray, about five at a time.

- Bake spring rolls for 3–4 minutes, turning a few times. When done, drain on kitchen paper.

- Serve with chilli sauce.

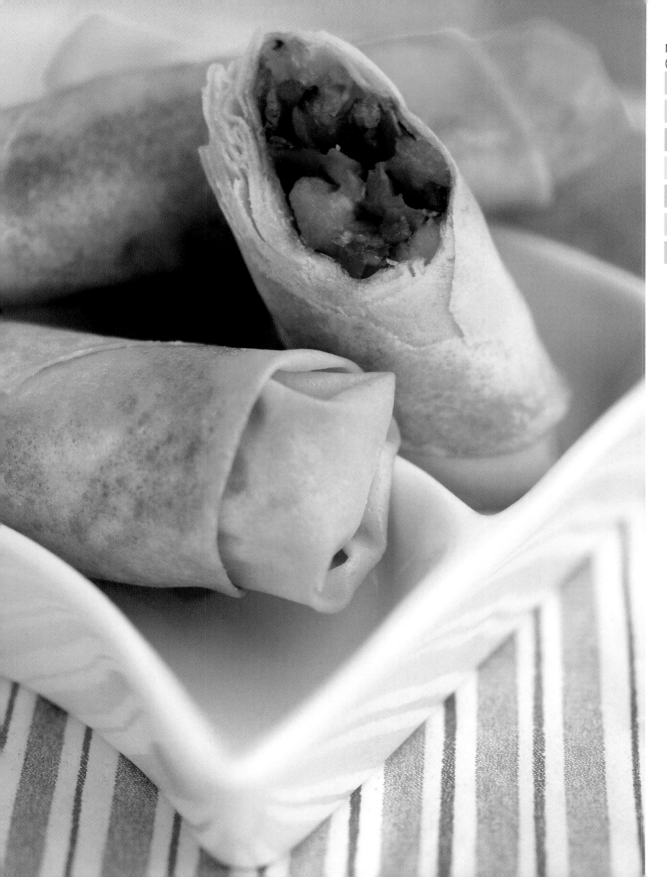

Nutrient Analysis
(per serving):

Calories: 62

Carbohydrates: 4 g

Total Fat: 2 g

Cholesterol: 24 mg

Protein: 6 g

Fibre: 1 g

Sodium: 236 mg

Nutrient Analysis
(per serving):

Calories: 118

Carbohydrates: 0 g

Total Fat: 9 g

Cholesterol: 52 mg

Protein: 9 g

Fibre: 0 g

Sodium: 384 mg

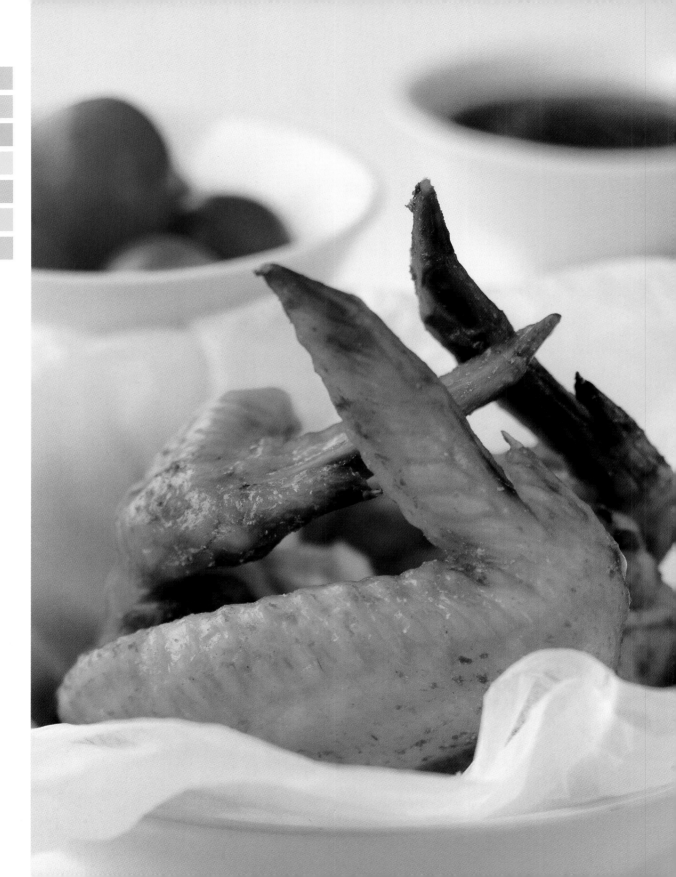

UN-FRIEDCHICKENWINGS

Nick's culinary jottings: Chicken wings, believe it or not, are the fattiest parts of a chicken (Indra nods her head in agreement). Hard to believe, but true! It is still beyond me how many people just love to eat chicken wings. Nevertheless, I have concocted this un-fried version that serves its purpose as a delightful snack.

Preparation time	: 10 minutes
Cooking time	: 15 minutes (includes steaming and baking)
Serves 3	

Method

- Season chicken with powders, tomato sauce, salt and pepper. Leave to marinate for a couple of hours.

- Steam marinated chicken for 4–5 minutes, then drain well.

- Preheat oven to 180°C (350°F). Heat baking tray.

- Remove tray from oven and apply spray oil. Arrange chicken on tray, then apply spray oil over top.

- Bake chicken for 8–10 minutes, turning every few minutes until done.

Ingredients

Chicken wings	6
Curry powder	2 tsp
Ground coriander (cilantro)	1 tsp
Tomato sauce	1 Tbsp
Salt and pepper	to taste
Spray oil	

CHAPLIKEBABS

Nick's culinary jottings: Originally, *chapli* kebabs were fried in tallow, which is lamb or beef fat. Being health conscious, however, we'll stick to our spray oil. Now, *chapli* literally means "slipper" and the kebabs were so named because in northern Pakistan, they were made large and flat and actually looked like sandals. If you are a heavy meat eater, then you are welcome to make your kebab quite that big. If not, then mould it into whatever shape and size you like.

Preparation time : 20 minutes
Cooking time : 20–30 minutes
Serves 4

Ingredients

Minced lean beef	500 g
Onions	250 g, peeled and coarsely chopped
Tomatoes	2, cubed
Green chillies	4, seeded and minced
Red chilli	1, seeded and minced
Cumin seeds	1 Tbsp, toasted in a dry pan and lightly crushed
Coriander (cilantro) seeds	1 Tbsp, toasted in a dry pan and lightly crushed
Garam masala	1 tsp
Chapati (*atta*) flour	60 g
Garlic paste	1 tsp
Ginger powder	1/2 tsp
Eggs	2, fried into an omelette, then finely sliced
Salt	to taste
Spray oil	3 squirts
Lemon juice	1 Tbsp

Method

- Except spray oil and lemon juice, combine all other ingredients in a bowl. Leave to marinate for about 1 hour.

- Shape combined ingredients into flattish shapes of your choice. Remember that they will not be deep-fried and large pieces are likely to break into bits as a result, so keep them manageable.

- Apply spray oil onto a pan. Heat pan slightly on stove. In the meantime, preheat oven to around 100°C (225°F) and line a baking try with tin foil.

- Add kebab pieces to pan. Move them around so they cook evenly.

- When kebabs are more or less cooked, transfer them to lined tray and cover with more foil. Place tray in oven and let kebabs cook further in their own juices until it is time to serve.

- Sprinkle on lemon juice just before serving. Alternatively, serve with lemon wedges on the side.

Note: If unavailable, chapati flour can be made by combining equal parts of wholemeal (wholewheat) flour and plain (all-purpose) flour. *Garam masala* is a powdered spice mixture commonly used in Indian cooking.

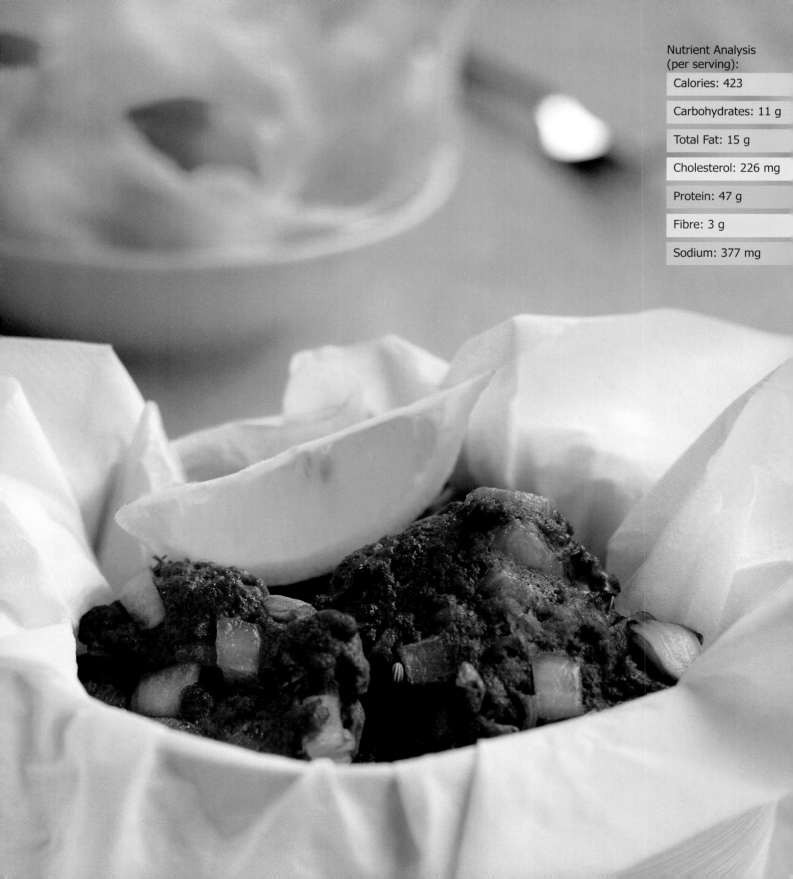

Nutrient Analysis
(per serving):

Calories: 423

Carbohydrates: 11 g

Total Fat: 15 g

Cholesterol: 226 mg

Protein: 47 g

Fibre: 3 g

Sodium: 377 mg

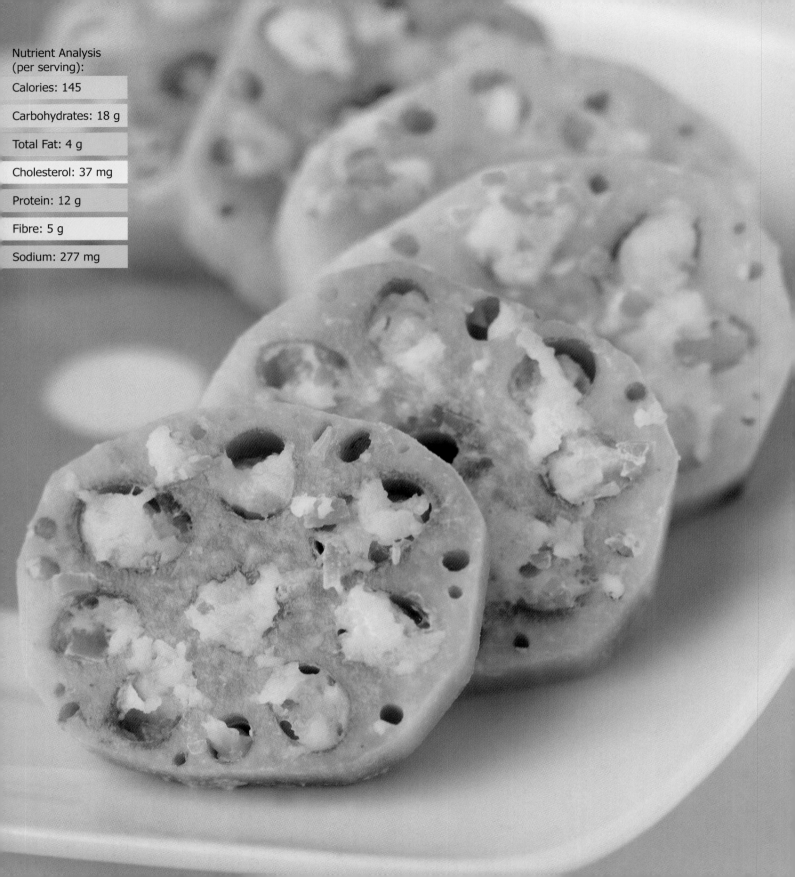

Nutrient Analysis
(per serving):

Calories: 145

Carbohydrates: 18 g

Total Fat: 4 g

Cholesterol: 37 mg

Protein: 12 g

Fibre: 5 g

Sodium: 277 mg

STUFFED LOTUS ROOT

Nick's culinary jottings: This is not an easy recipe but the results will leave your family or guests in awe. The Asian water lily root is most often used in soups. It can also be used in stir-fries, however, and even in a salad. This is after all a root, so please clean it thoroughly as you will find remnants of mud. In the market, try to find the ones with both ends sealed. With this recipe, you will also learn to make your own fish balls which are much better than the ones bought.

Preparation time : 30–40 minutes
Cooking time : 60 minutes (includes boiling of lotus root)

Serves 5

Method

- Soak lotus root pieces in water for several minutes to clean. Then, boil pieces in some water. Add a little salt to taste. When almost done, drain pieces and set aside.

- Blend (process) mackerel until paste-like, then transfer to a bowl. Rub some salt water onto hands before handling fish paste to avoid a sticky mess.

- Season paste with sesame seed oil, fish sauce, sugar and pepper to taste. Mix in carrot and onion. Add corn flour to bind paste.

- Fill cavities of lotus root pieces with fish paste. Use a chopstick to ensure paste is packed as tightly as possible.

- Steam lotus root for about 20 minutes or until soft like a cooked potato. Serve sliced.

Note: Blender (processor) can also be cleaned of fish paste using salt water.

Ingredients

Lotus root (*leen ngau*)	40-cm piece, peeled and cut at each segment
Mackerel fish fillet	250 g
Sesame seed oil	1 tsp
Fish sauce	1 tsp
Sugar	1/2 tsp
Finely chopped carrot	1 Tbsp
Finely chopped onion	1 Tbsp
Corn flour (cornstarch)	1 tsp
Salt and pepper	to taste

Nicholas

We have salad days, and we just don't. I know sometimes I can devour a whole box of salad without any problems but at other times, I will be grumbling and complaining about how bitter it is and all. Salads can be really insipid if they are not appropriately jazzed up. Asians are so used to food rich with spices and ingredients that bring together vibrant flavours that eating plain leaves becomes something of a challenge, and something quite short-term.

I have created a few salads that won't make me grumble if it is served. You know, in Asia, we are spoilt for choice, with so many ingredients to make our salad dressings so much better than the usual mayonnaise or other oil-based dressings. Remember that healthy eating is also about eating with enjoyment, so if you don't enjoy it, you will never carry on eating in a more nutritious way.

Indra

Honestly, the most recommended way to eat your vegetables is raw as the antioxidants aren't destroyed by high heat applied during cooking. In fact, experts are uncovering many wonderful health aspects related to eating certain vegetables and herbs. Obviously, certain vegetables don't taste so great when they're raw. For those that do, making them into a salad is simply a glorious nutritional boost to your daily diet!

The high-fat part of the salad is usually the dressing or salad cream, of which the main ingredient is oil. The reality, however, is that salads taste quite blah without it, so by all means use some salad dressing, but be light-handed with it. A little goes a long way in flavouring your salad.

Kitchen hygiene needs to be strictly practised when preparing salads. Be mindful of not using the same chopping board to cut vegetables after you've cut meat. This advice sounds simple enough but is usually overlooked. No point eating healthily if you're going to end up poisoning yourself.

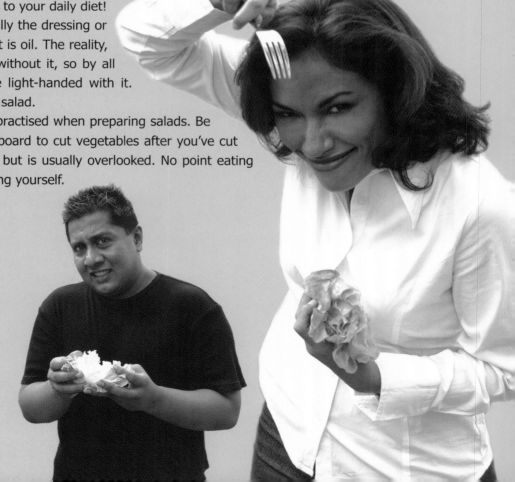

SALADS

PRAWN WITH PIQUANT SHERRY DRESSING

Preparation time : 20 minutes
Cooking time : 5 minutes
Serves 2

Nick's culinary jottings: This prawn salad is fairly easy to make and not as heavy as most prawn salads I know.

Ingredients

Fresh dill	1 tsp
Lemon juice	1 Tbsp
Castor (superfine) sugar	1/2 tsp
Sherry	60 ml
Medium–large prawns (shrimps)	200 g, peeled, deveined, boiled and soaked in iced water
Plain low-fat yoghurt	60 g
Coarse ground mustard	2 tsp
Ground coriander (cilantro)	1 tsp
Ground black pepper	1 tsp

Method

- To make marinade, combine dill, lemon juice, sugar and 40 ml sherry. Add prawns and leave to marinate in refrigerator.

- To make dressing, combine remaining sherry, yoghurt, mustard, coriander and pepper. Mix well and set aside.

- Serve prawns alongside your favourite vegetable. Drizzle dressing over the top.

Note: For a more fanciful serving suggestion, cut 2 iceberg lettuce leaves into circles with scissors, then line a plate with each. Arrange prawns on top of lettuce and drizzle on dressing. Sprinkle on minced fresh dill and julienned lemon rind for garnish.

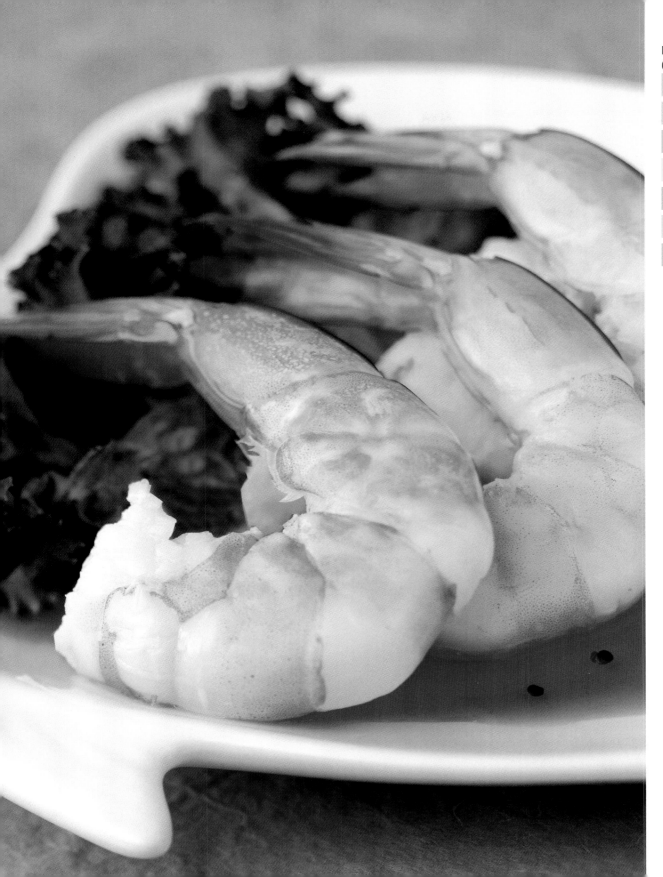

Nutrient Analysis
(per serving):

Calories: 168

Carbohydrates: 7 g

Total Fat: 3 g

Cholesterol: 154 mg

Protein: 23 g

Fibre: 1 g

Sodium: 170 mg

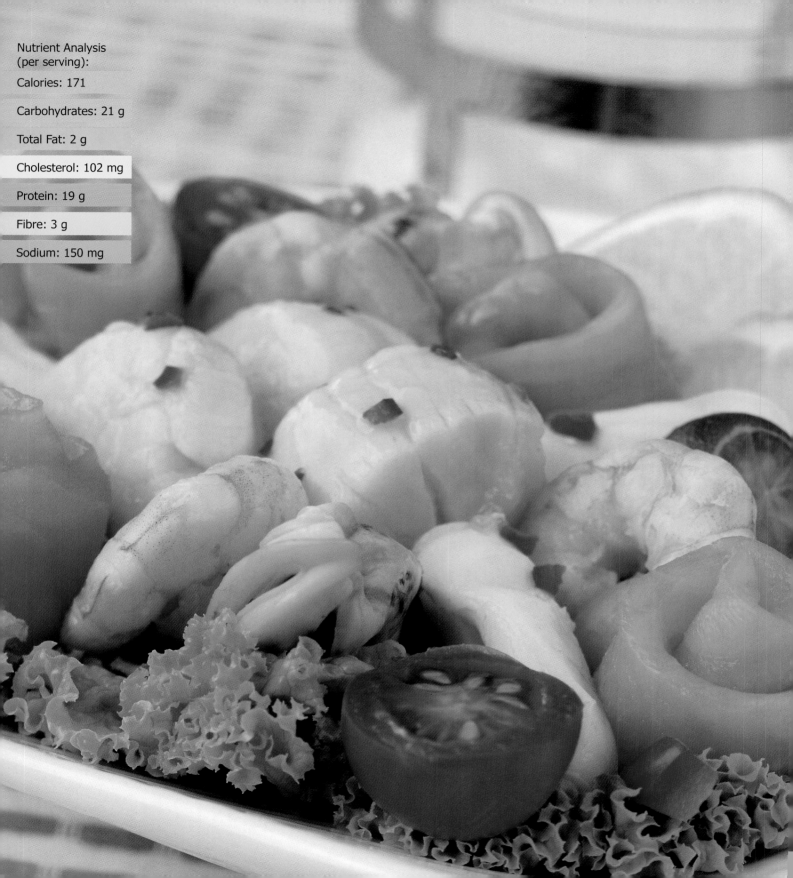

Nutrient Analysis
(per serving):

Calories: 171

Carbohydrates: 21 g

Total Fat: 2 g

Cholesterol: 102 mg

Protein: 19 g

Fibre: 3 g

Sodium: 150 mg

KOKONDA (SEAFOOD SALAD)

Nick's culinary jottings: This is an uncooked seafood salad originating from Fiji. The dish was made by my Fijian friend, Mereiseini Waibuta. The Fijian recipe is eaten with coconut cream. However, seeing as we're trying to maintain a slick and slender body, we will look for other options. Hygiene and freshness is of utmost importance here.

Preparation time : 20 minutes
Serves 4

Method

- In a large bowl, combine all seafood, garlic, lemon and lime juices, sugar and salt. Mix thoroughly. Cover bowl with cling film (plastic wrap). Refrigerate overnight.

- The next day, just before serving, strain excess juice from seafood and reserve. Add to seafood onion, chilli, capsicum and tomatoes. Mix well.

- Arrange mixed ingredients on top of lettuce leaves. Add a little juice for dressing. Sprinkle on some freshly cracked pepper if desired.

- Serve with a dollop of yoghurt if preferred.

Note: Do not say anything to your guests about the seafood being uncooked in the traditional sense because it usually makes everyone go squeamish.

Ingredients

Small squid tubes	100 g
Prawns (shrimps)	50 g, peeled and deveined
Tuna or salmon steaks	100 g, thinly sliced
Mussels	10, shucked
Scallops	10
Garlic	3 cloves, peeled and minced
Lemon juice	250 ml
Kalamansi or other lime juice	125 ml
Sugar	1 tsp or more to taste
Salt	1 pinch
Onion	1, large, peeled and minced
Red chilli	1, seeded and minced
Red capsicum (sweet bell pepper)	1, cut into small squares
Cherry tomatoes	1 punnet, each halved
Cos (romaine) lettuce leaves	
Freshly cracked black pepper (optional)	
Plain low-fat yoghurt (optional)	

MANGOKERABU

Nick's culinary jottings: It's funny how eating mango *kerabu* in a restaurant can give you onion breath! Although it's a mango salad, these thrifty restaurants put more onion than mango, a practice that is simply shocking considering mangoes are available practically all year round in the tropics. In short, then, make your own so that you can be generous with all the luscious ingredients. It's really very easy, you know.

Preparation time : 15 minutes
Serves 5

Ingredients

Mango (variety of your choice)	2, large and slightly ripe
Lime juice	125 ml
Brown sugar	2 tsp
Fish sauce	2 Tbsp
Salt	1 pinch
Onion	1, large, peeled and thinly sliced
Bird's eye chillies (*cili padi*)	2, minced
Dried prawns (shrimps)	2 Tbsp, dry-fried and coarsely ground
Torch ginger bud (*bunga kantan*)	1 stalk, julienned
Kaffir lime leaves	2, julienned
Roasted unsalted peanuts (groundnuts)	75 g, coarsely ground

Method

- Peel mangoes, then slice off fleshy parts on either side of seed. Julienne mango flesh.

- To make dressing, combine lime juice, brown sugar, fish sauce and salt. Set aside.

- Except peanuts, combine remaining ingredients. Add dressing and stir to mix thoroughly.

- Sprinkle on peanuts and serve immediately.

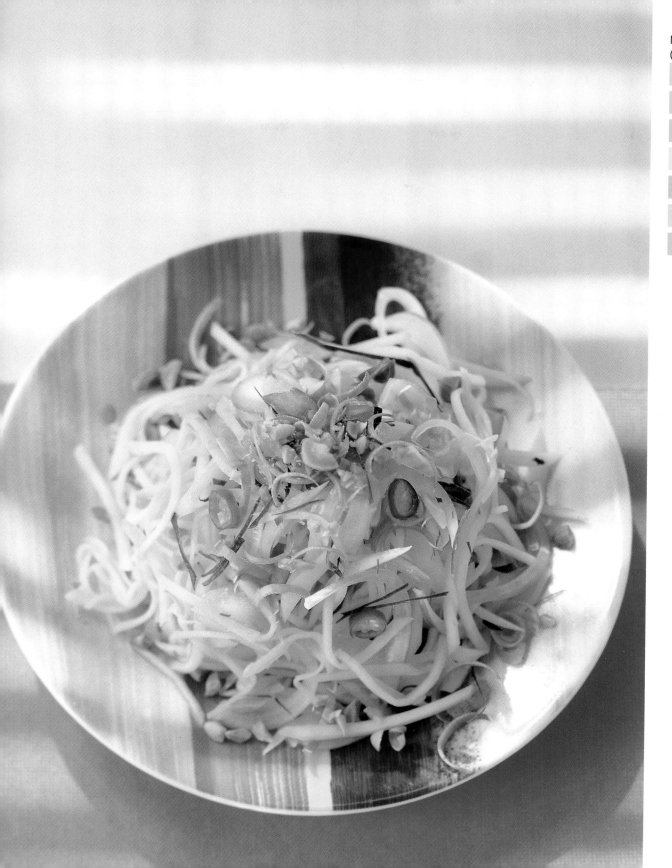

Nutrient Analysis
(per serving):

Calories: 170

Carbohydrates: 21 g

Total Fat: 8 g

Cholesterol: 2 mg

Protein: 7 g

Fibre: 3 g

Sodium: 158 mg

Nutrient Analysis
(per serving):

Calories: 373

Carbohydrates: 74 g

Total Fat: 1 g

Cholesterol: 0 mg

Protein: 18 g

Fibre: 12 g

Sodium: 182 mg

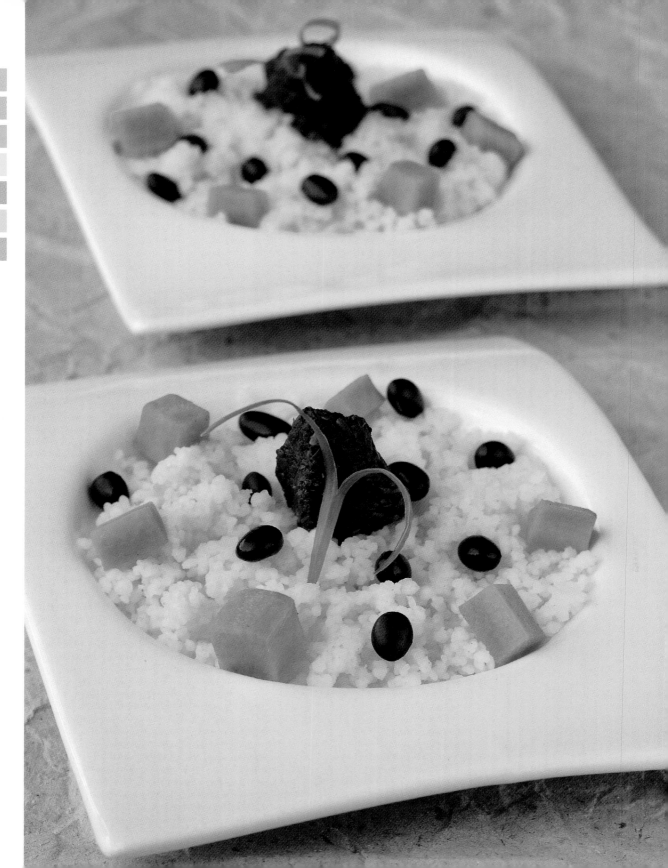

COUSCOUS AND BLACK BEAN SALAD

Nick's culinary jottings: This recipe is high in Omega 3 fatty acids (yes, the healthy kind) because of the inclusion of black beans and spinach. A one-pot wonder, this recipe can be eaten hot or cold, as a starter or even main course, after you throw in some extra vegetables.

Preparation time : 30 minutes
Cooking time : 60 minutes
Serves 4

Method

- In a pot, sauté onions over low heat with 125 ml stock until fragrant.

- Add remaining stock and carrots. Leave to boil for about 5 minutes or until carrots are partially cooked. Add fennel.

- Add couscous, black pepper, cumin and salt to taste. Leave to boil until couscous has puffed up.

- Transfer sufficient couscous to individual serving plates. Sprinkle on beans. Add a dollop of spinach to each plate. Garnish with spring onions.

- Alternatively, add black beans and spinach to cooked couscous in the pot. Then, add more stock if you prefer it watery. Simmer for a few minutes more. Mix in coriander leaves if used.

- Serve hot or cold.

Ingredients

Onions	2, large, peeled and cubed
Stock	500 ml
Chopped carrots	150 g
Fennel	1 tsp, toasted in a dry pan
Couscous	245 g
Cracked black pepper	1 tsp
Ground cumin	1 tsp
Salt	to taste
Black beans	1 cup, boiled until just done and not mushy soft
Cooked spinach	90 g, chopped
Julienned spring onions (scallions)	
Coriander (cilantro) leaves (optional)	30 g

LENTILSALAD

Nick's culinary jottings: This is one of the easiest salads to make as all you do is boil the lentils and kidney beans and everything else is just mixed in. Okay, of course there is some cutting up to do, but altogether it's not too bad.

Preparation time : 20 minutes (not including boiling of lentils)

Serves 4

Ingredients

Chickpeas	160 g, soaked and boiled until done
Skinned *masoor* dhal	80 g, soaked and boiled until done; replaceable with red lentils
Kidney beans	100 g, soaked and boiled until done
Onion	1, large, peeled and minced
Celery	3 stalks, thinly sliced
Mint leaves	30 g, coarsely chopped
Red capsicum (sweet bell pepper)	1, seeded and cut into squares
Chilli flakes	1 tsp or more to taste
Toasted almond slivers	65 g

Dressing

Black pepper	1 tsp
Balsamic vinegar	3 Tbsp
Ground nutmeg	$^1/_2$ tsp
Wasabi paste	1 tsp or more to taste
Sugar	1 pinch
Lemon juice	to taste

Method

- Combine all dressing ingredients. Taste it to see if it is to your liking. If not, then adjust to taste. When done, set aside.

- In a bowl, combine all salad ingredients. Add dressing, then refrigerate. Serve as a cold starter or as a meal on its own on one of those lazy days.

- Try to consume salad in one sitting as it tastes better fresh.

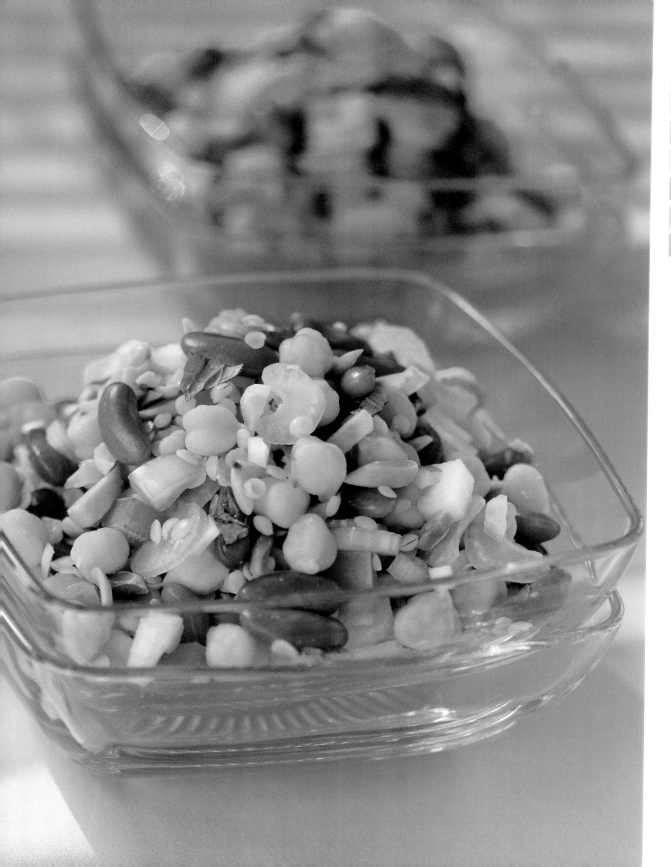

Nutrient Analysis
(per serving):

Calories: 496

Carbohydrates: 73 g

Total Fat: 13 g

Cholesterol: 0 mg

Protein: 28 g

Fibre: 28 g

Sodium: 89 mg

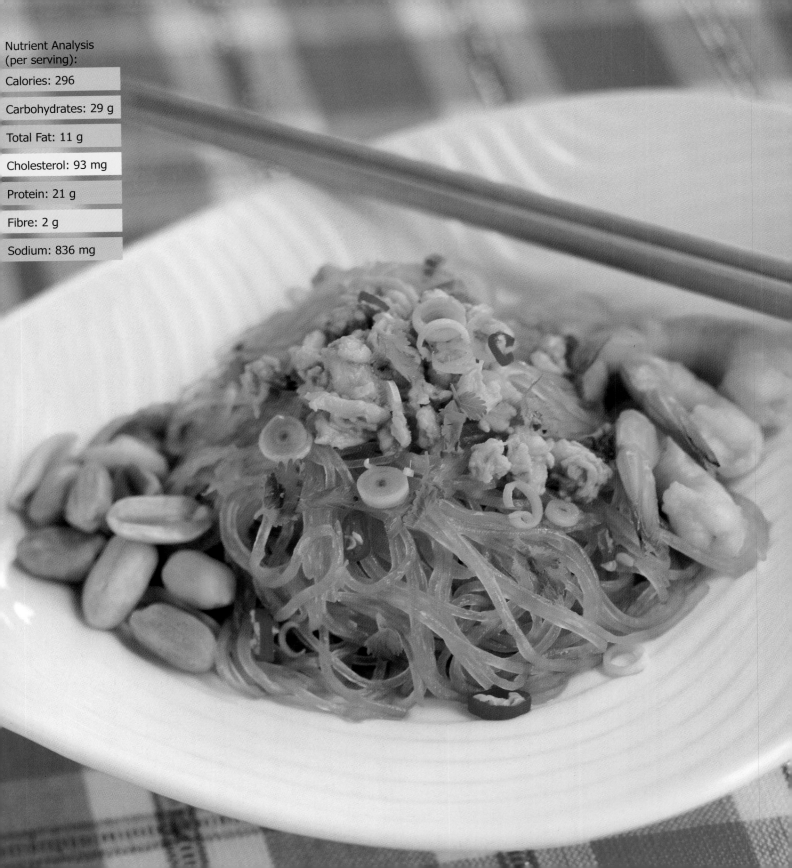

Nutrient Analysis
(per serving):

Calories: 296

Carbohydrates: 29 g

Total Fat: 11 g

Cholesterol: 93 mg

Protein: 21 g

Fibre: 2 g

Sodium: 836 mg

YAMWOONSEN(THAINOODLESALAD)

Nick's culinary jottings: I ate this salad in a Thai restaurant in Australia and absolutely fell in love with it. You have to eat it immediately after it is served or it will not be as tasty. It is so easy to make and actually rather healthy. Interestingly, if you do not boil the noodles properly, you will get air in your stomach, so cook it properly to prevent discomfort.

Preparation time : 20–30 minutes
Cooking time : 20 minutes
Serves 4

Method

- To make dressing, combine lemon juice, fish sauce and sugar. Toss noodles in dressing.

- Transfer noodles to centre of a serving platter. Arrange each of the remaining ingredients around noodles, like petals of a flower.

- To serve, set platter on dining table. Get everyone around the table to toss ingredients together in true *loh hei* style, i.e. each person uses his or her eating utensil, whether chopsticks or a fork, to help mix all the ingredients together by tossing toward the platter's centre.

- For a less messy serving suggestion, add onions, chillies, lemon grass and coriander to noodles after they have been tossed in dressing. Mix well, then portion noodles onto individual serving plates. Put a few prawns, some chicken and peanuts on the side of noodles. Garnish with more chilli, lemon grass and coriander if desired.

Note: *Loh hei* is something the Chinese say when they get ready to eat a raw fish dish available only during the Chinese New Year period. The dish, called *yu sang*, requires everyone at the table to stand and toss a large platter of various julienned ingredients together using their chopsticks. The belief is that the higher the food is tossed, the better everyone's luck will be in the coming year. Once thoroughly mixed, the diners will sit down to enjoy the fruit of their labour.

Ingredients

Lemon juice	125 ml
Fish sauce	2–3 Tbsp
Sugar	1 pinch
Glass noodles (*fun see*)	100 g, soaked and boiled until done
Onions	5–6, small, peeled and finely sliced
Bird's eye chillies (*cili padi*)	2–3, minced
Young lemon grass (*serai*)	1 stalk, finely sliced
Coriander (cilantro) leaves	1 sprig
Minced chicken	100 g, boiled and drained
Medium-sized prawns (shrimps)	200 g, peeled, deveined and boiled
Roasted unsalted peanuts (groundnuts)	75 g, the smaller variety is preferred

Nicholas

While many of us, myself included, are fussy when it comes to veggies, it is something we have to deal with. As kids, mum and dad were there to threaten us but with age, we tend to forget about veggies altogether, and for long periods of time at that. I know I went through that. In fact, one of my good friends, Angeline, still won't touch anything green. The next time I cook veggies for her, I will remember to dye them red.

In my years of cooking, I have found that making a dish look good also makes it go down well. This is because these days, people feast as much with their eyes and you know how first impressions are, so make your veggies as interesting as possible.

Indra

Poor vegetables — people just never give them enough credit. They are always second fiddle to a meat or seafood dish that is usually the star of the dinner table. Think roast chicken and vegetables, or Ipoh chicken rice and bean sprouts. Vegetables are like always the bridesmaid and never the bride!

The true power nutrients in vegetables and fruit lie in their unique colour pigmentation. Differently coloured veggies contain different types of antioxidants that researchers have found are able to combat free radical cell damage in your body. Free radicals are molecules that have lost their partners and are on a quest to look for cells to latch onto to complete themselves. But in so doing, they actually cause damage to your otherwise healthy cells. Eating plenty of vegetables and fruit daily, then, helps your body's natural defence mechanism.

Make sure that you include veggies that are purple/red (aubergine, red cabbage, etc.); yellow/orange (pumpkin, squash, carrot, etc.); and white (turnip, radish, etc.). Think rainbow, really — if it's not colourful, it's not enough!

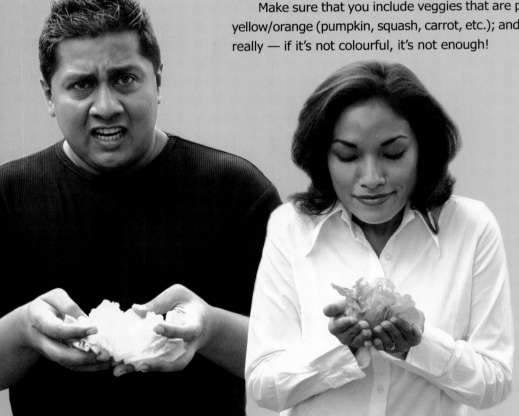

COOKED VEGETABLES

KANGKUNGBELACAN

Nick's culinary jottings: Kangkung or water convolvulus is one of the easiest vegetables to grow and it is high in nourishment. *Kangkung belacan* is an all-time Malaysian favourite and although the vegetable is among the easiest to cook, it is frequently ordered when eating out.

Preparation time : 20 minutes
Cooking time : 10 minutes
Serves 5

Ingredients

Garlic	1 clove, peeled and minced
Onion	1, small, peeled and minced
Red chilli	1, seeded and sliced
Spray oil	3 squirts
Water convolvulus (*kangkung*)	1 kg, washed and drained several times to remove sand and grit
Dried prawn (shrimp) paste (*belacan*) granules	2 tsp
Sugar	1 pinch
Corn flour (cornstarch)	2 tsp, mixed with a little water to make thickener
Salt	to taste

Method

- Heat a dry pan. When hot, add garlic, onion and chilli. Spray on oil. Sauté until ingredients are lightly brown.

- Add vegetables. Sprinkle on dried prawn paste granules. Stir well until vegetables are done to your liking. You may like it a little crunchier or softer, so respectively shorten or extend cooking time.

- Season to taste with sugar and salt, then add corn flour mixture. When liquid thickens, dish out and serve immediately.

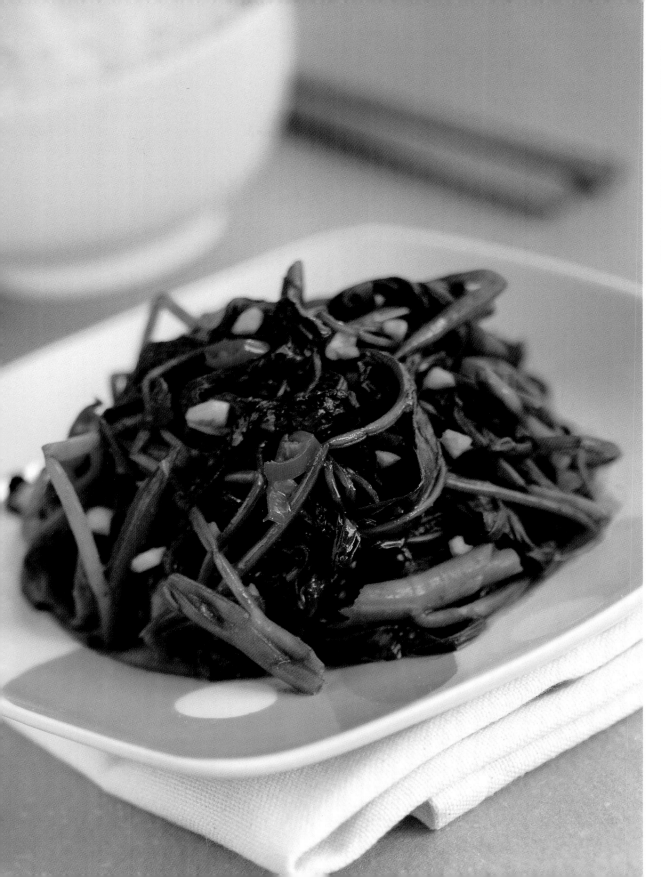

Nutrient Analysis
(per serving):

Calories: 71

Carbohydrates: 9 g

Total Fat: 0 g

Cholesterol: 0 mg

Protein: 6 g

Fibre: 2 g

Sodium: 282 mg

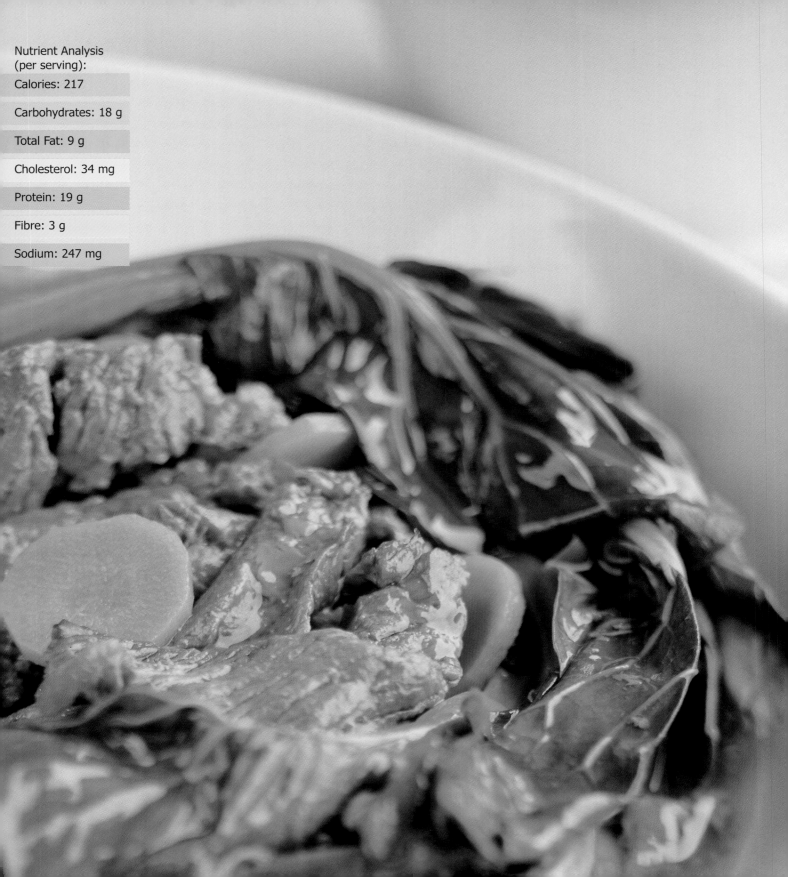

Nutrient Analysis
(per serving):

Calories: 217

Carbohydrates: 18 g

Total Fat: 9 g

Cholesterol: 34 mg

Protein: 19 g

Fibre: 3 g

Sodium: 247 mg

KAILAN BEEF

Nick's culinary jottings: I like this dish because it is a vegetable dish with enough meat. This is another favourite that is often ordered when eating out and, yet, is so easy to make at home.

Preparation time : 20 minutes
Cooking time : 10–15 minutes
Serves 4

Method

- Bring stock to the boil. Add garlic, ginger and beef. Simmer over low heat for about 20 minutes or until beef is tender. Add carrot. Simmer for 5 minutes more.

- Increase heat and add kale. Season to taste, then add corn flour mixture. When liquid thickens, dish out.

- Serve with rice.

♟ Note: Chinese kale is sometimes also known as Chinese broccoli. To choose young kale, look at the stems; thick stems indicate that the vegetable is old.

Ingredients

Stock	250 ml
Garlic	1 clove, peeled and minced
Ginger	1 small knob, peeled and finely sliced
Sirloin steak	200 g, thinly sliced, then marinated with a little light soy sauce, ground pepper, tenderiser and a pinch of sugar
Carrot	1, peeled and thinly sliced
Young Chinese kale (*kailan*)	500 g, leave stalks whole only for better presentation
Salt and pepper	to taste
Corn flour (cornstarch)	2 tsp, mixed with a little water to make thickener

ROASTEDVEGETABLES

Nick's culinary jottings: This is a really easy recipe that can be done heaps in advance. Vegetables, like meat, can be marinated and kept in the refrigerator before you leave home in the morning and when you get home, stick it in the oven, take your shower and come down to a nice plateful of roasted vegetables. If you want it faster, lightly parboil the vegetables before roasting. It is necessary to use hard vegetables or they will become mushy and yucky. Gosh, I think that rhymes. Next book... poetry?!

Preparation time : 20 minutes
Cooking time : 30–40 minutes
Serves 2

Ingredients

Carrots	2, large, peeled if desired and cut any way you like
Potatoes	2, large, peeled if desired and cut into large cubes
Pumpkin	1, small, peeled, seeded and cut into cubes
Cauliflower	1/2 a medium-size head, cut into large florets
Dried rosemary	1 tsp
Dried oregano	1 pinch
Curry powder	1 pinch
Salt and pepper	to taste
Spray oil	

Method

- Parboil carrots, potatoes and pumpkin in some water, with a little salt. After 10 minutes, add cauliflower. When ingredients are half-cooked, drain and remove to a large bowl.

- Season parboiled ingredients with rosemary, oregano, curry powder and salt and pepper to taste. Cover bowl with cling film (plastic wrap). Leave to marinate in refrigerator. Alternatively, roast vegetables immediately after seasoning.

- Preheat oven to 200°C (400°F).

- Transfer vegetables to a baking tray. Spray on one coat of oil, then bake until done. Check with a skewer. If the potatoes are done, then everything else should be fine. Serve and eat hot.

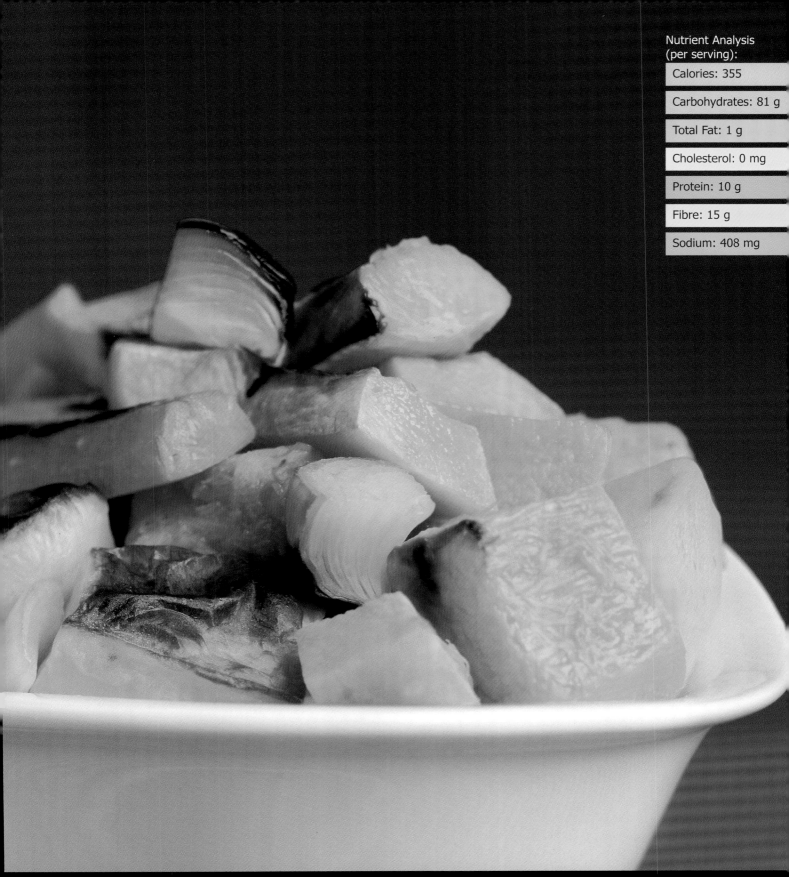

Nutrient Analysis
(per serving):

Calories: 192

Carbohydrates: 25 g

Total Fat: 6 g

Cholesterol: 0 mg

Protein: 20 g

Fibre: 4 g

Sodium: 251 mg

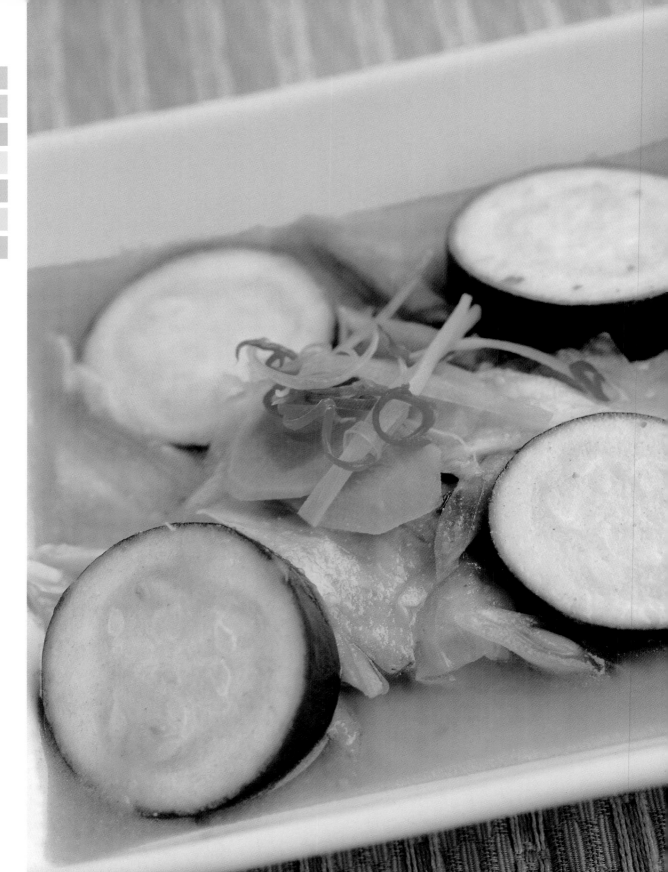

SAYURLODEH

Nick's culinary jottings: *Sayur lodeh* is a form of curried mixed vegetables, with bits of Indonesian and Malaysia and even Portuguese flavours thrown in. It's not really a delicacy but each year, the day after Ramadan, we would go to Aunty Shina's (she passed on in 1992) to savour this dish. To this day, her mother still makes the best *sayur lodeh*, i.e. with all the thrills and frills of coconut milk. Once a year, I guess, is okay. The vegetables in this dish are usually boiled until they are rather mushy or pulpy but here, for health reasons, we won't. We need the fibres okay!

Preparation time : 30 minutes
Cooking time : 30–40 minutes
Serves 5

Method

- In a pot, combine stock and rice milk. Bring to the boil.
- Add onion, garlic, galangal, turmeric, bay leaves, lemon grass and dried prawns. Simmer for about 10 minutes or until fragrant.
- Add choco and simmer until soft.
- Add beans, cabbage, carrot and fermented soybean cake. Boil for 10 minutes.
- Add chillies, sugar and salt to taste. Lastly, add soy milk and bring to the boil over high heat.

Note: Choco is also known as vegetable pear, chayote, and *fut sau kwa* or "buddha's hand gourd" in Cantonese. If unavailable, use 180 g courgette (zucchini), thickly sliced, instead.

Ingredients

Stock	250 ml
Rice milk	250 ml
Onion	1, peeled and finely sliced
Garlic	1, peeled and minced
Galangal (*lengkuas*)	1 small knob, about 1 Tbsp if pounded
Turmeric (*kunyit*)	1 small knob, pounded until fine
Bay leaves (*daun salam*)	2
Lemon grass (*serai*)	2 stalks, bruised
Dried prawns (shrimps)(*ha mai*)	1 Tbsp, toasted in a dry pan and pounded until fine
Choco	1, cut into large cubes
French beans	200 g, cut diagonally into 2-cm lengths
Cabbage	200 g, cut into small, uniform chunks
Carrot	1, large, peeled and sliced
Fermented soybean cake (*tempe*)	200 g, wrapped in foil and roasted at 180°C (350°F) for 10–15 minutes, then cut into bite-size cubes
Green chillies	2, halved lengthways (lengthwise) and seeded
Red chilli	1, halved lengthways (lengthwise) and seeded
Sugar	1 pinch
Salt	to taste
Soy milk	250 ml

LOTUSROOTSOUP

Nick's culinary jottings: My mother always said that eating Asian water lily root, or lotus root, is like eating meat, and she is so right. Cut it into nice chunky pieces, boil them for a few hours and the resulting flavour is just divine.

Preparation time : 30 minutes
Cooking time : 90 minutes
Serves 4

Ingredients

Water	1.5 litres
Lotus root (*leen ngau*)	1 kg, peeled, sliced and thoroughly cleaned
Chicken bones	1 kg
Dried Chinese red dates (*hung cho*)	100 g
Chinese wolfberries (*gei chi*)	100 g
Sugar	1 pinch
Salt and pepper	to taste

Method

- In a large pot, bring water, lotus root and bones to the boil. Simmer for about 40 minutes.

- Add dates and wolfberries. Season to taste with sugar, salt and pepper.

- Simmer some more until lotus root is biteable. Serve hot.

- This recipe can be frozen for future consumption as the lotus root slices will not become mushy.

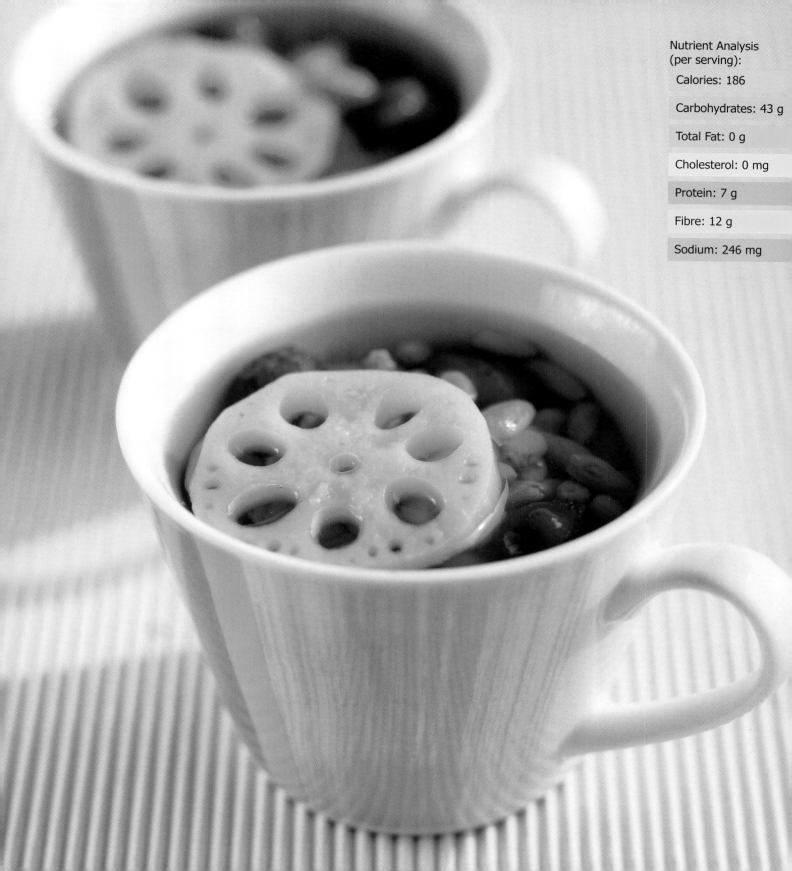

Nutrient Analysis
(per serving):

Calories: 186

Carbohydrates: 43 g

Total Fat: 0 g

Cholesterol: 0 mg

Protein: 7 g

Fibre: 12 g

Sodium: 246 mg

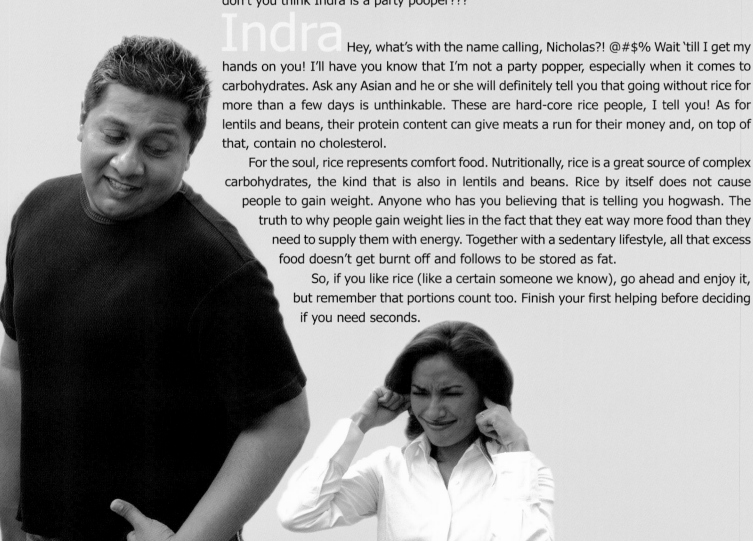

Nicholas

Rice, the mere aroma of rice is enough to make me go all funny. I love my rice, I love it plain, I love it any way its presented. In fact, most of my foreign friends came to realise how nice rice can be simply because I used to do so many things with it. Just add a bit of this and a bit of that and a whole new creation is made.

Lentils, on the other hand, I hated as a kid, and I am sure I have mentioned it more than once in this book. I came to appreciate them only much later on in life and after Vaea Matapo, a friend from Tahiti, showed me how delicious they could become in her well-loved ham hock stew. It is just as well that they are healthy.

Rice and lentils, however, are also carbohydrates, and for all the things we hear about them these days, we should be careful how much of them we consume. I am sure Indra will have a few things to say about this, in any case. Hmmm, what do you think, or is it just me, don't you think Indra is a party pooper???

Indra

Hey, what's with the name calling, Nicholas?! @#$% Wait 'till I get my hands on you! I'll have you know that I'm not a party popper, especially when it comes to carbohydrates. Ask any Asian and he or she will definitely tell you that going without rice for more than a few days is unthinkable. These are hard-core rice people, I tell you! As for lentils and beans, their protein content can give meats a run for their money and, on top of that, contain no cholesterol.

For the soul, rice represents comfort food. Nutritionally, rice is a great source of complex carbohydrates, the kind that is also in lentils and beans. Rice by itself does not cause people to gain weight. Anyone who has you believing that is telling you hogwash. The truth to why people gain weight lies in the fact that they eat way more food than they need to supply them with energy. Together with a sedentary lifestyle, all that excess food doesn't get burnt off and follows to be stored as fat.

So, if you like rice (like a certain someone we know), go ahead and enjoy it, but remember that portions count too. Finish your first helping before deciding if you need seconds.

RICE AND LENTILS

LEMONRICE

Nick's culinary jottings: The first time I ate this rice dish was at a cooking demonstration. I was with a good friend of mine, Mrs. Manju Saigal. I took one spoonful and after that, I simply could not stop shovelling the rice into my mouth. It was just divine! Try it with the lentils or dhal you have on hand, it is a complete meal.

Preparation time : 15 minutes
Cooking time : 15 minutes
Serves 6

Ingredients

Basmati rice	410 g
Mustard seeds	2 tsp
Spray oil	2 squirts
Green lentils	80 g, soaked
Red lentils	80 g, soaked
Yellow lentils	80 g, soaked
Water	500 ml (you may not need all of it)
Asafoetida	1 Tbsp or more to taste
Ground turmeric (*kunyit*)	2 tsp
Fresh curry leaves	15 g
Lemon or lime juice	to taste
Salt	to taste
Skinless raw peanuts (groundnuts)	75 g, split and dry-roasted in oven
Green chillies	5–6, thinly sliced
Coriander (cilantro) leaves	60 g, coarsely chopped

Method

- Cook rice with sufficient water and a little salt. Undo lumps in cooled cooked rice, then set aside.

- Heat a dry pan. Toast mustard seeds without burning. When seeds start to pop, apply spray oil.

- Add all lentils and stir through. Add a little water and let simmer for a few minutes. Lentils do not have to be cooked; add asafoetida and turmeric. Stir through.

- Add curry leaves and stir to mix. Add lemon or lime juice and salt to taste.

- Over low heat, add rice and mix well. Add peanuts and chillies. If it is dry, add a little water. Adjust to taste with more salt or lemon juice if needed.

- To serve, garnish with coriander. Eat hot or at room temperature.

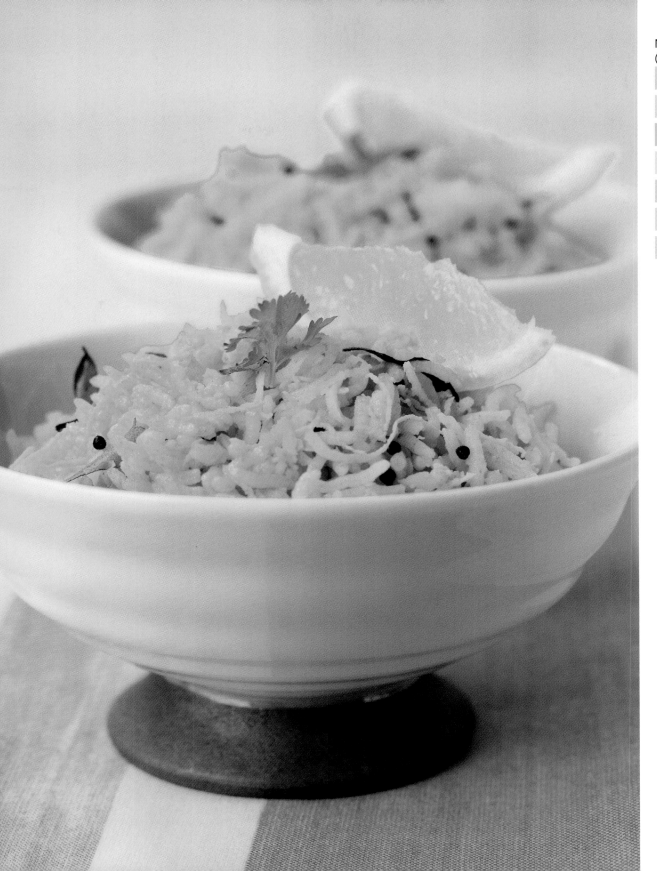

Nutrient Analysis
(per serving):

Calories: 479

Carbohydrates: 83 g

Total Fat: 7 g

Cholesterol: 0 mg

Protein: 22 g

Fibre: 17 g

Sodium: 109 mg

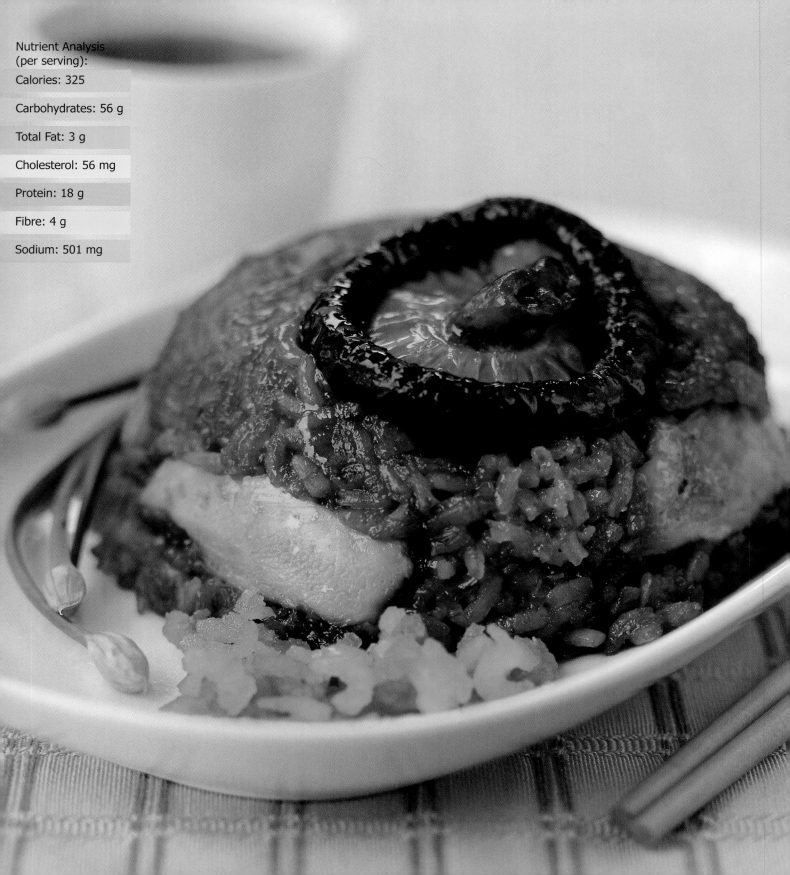

Nutrient Analysis
(per serving):

Calories: 325

Carbohydrates: 56 g

Total Fat: 3 g

Cholesterol: 56 mg

Protein: 18 g

Fibre: 4 g

Sodium: 501 mg

LOHMAIKAI

Nick's culinary jottings: Loh mai kai or glutinous rice and chicken was a firm favourite when we were kids but when we grew up, we became a little apprehensive because of the amount of fat it contains, from the pork fat in the Chinese sausages *(lap cheong)* to the copious amounts of oil used to cook the dish and consequently absorbed by the rice. If you don't believe me, buy one from the shop and refrigerate it for a few hours. You will find it almost entirely covered in solid grease. Our version here is not so oily and surely not so fatty. Try it ok?

Method

- Put rice in a large container, then steam over high heat.

- In a wok or nonstick pan, quickly sear chicken with garlic and onion. Then, add stock and leave to boil for a few minutes. Add dried prawns and simmer for 2–3 minutes more.

- Add remaining ingredients. Do not cook for much longer as you need sufficient liquid for cooking the rice later.

- Pour chicken and liquid over steaming rice. Stir well to mix. If rice does not puff up enough in time, add more stock.

- Steam until rice is cooked through.

- To serve, garnish with one or more of the following: chopped spring onions (scallions) or chives, roasted unsalted peanuts (groundnuts) and sliced red chillies. If preferred, add some dried prawns (shrimps) that have been soaked and then toasted until crispy on the side.

Preparation time : 30 minutes
Cooking time : 60 minutes
Serves 6

Ingredients

Glutinous rice	300 g, soaked in lightly salted water, then washed and drained
Chicken thigh fillets	250 g, cut into strips, then seasoned with 1 Tbsp dark soy sauce, 1 tsp five-spice powder and 1 pinch sugar
Garlic	2–3 cloves, peeled and minced
Onion	1/2, large, peeled and minced
Stock	750 ml
Dried prawns (shrimps) (*ha mai*)	50 g, soaked
Dried Chinese mushrooms	8–10, boiled, stems discarded and halved if desired
Five-spice powder	1 tsp
Dark soy sauce	3–4 Tbsp or more to taste
Light soy sauce	1 Tbsp
Sugar	2 tsp
Sesame seed oil	2 tsp
Salt and pepper	to taste

CHICKENRICEBALLS

Nick's culinary jottings: Malacca is the birthplace of chicken rice balls. I quite liked them simply because they were novel. I do remember, however, looking at the plate and thinking how empty it looked and frankly, I was not the only one. There were just some chicken pieces and five rice balls. Boring, I thought, so I decided to do my own little concoction to make it a squarer meal — more veggies and other delicious stuff.

Preparation time : 30 minutes
Cooking time : 60 minutes (does not include stock-boiling)
Serves 6

Ingredients

Calrose short grain rice	555 g, washed and drained
Chicken stock*	1 recipe
Chicken thigh fillets	5, skinned and excess fat trimmed, then marinated with a little light soy sauce and ground pepper
Salt	1 pinch or more to taste
Tomatoes	2–3, cut into wedges
Cucumbers	1–2, peeled if desired and cut any way you like
Bean sprouts	100 g
Coriander (cilantro)	2–3 sprigs, roughly chopped
Spring onions (scallions)	

Chicken stock

Chicken bones	500 g
Ginger	50 g, peeled and sliced
Garlic	3–4 cloves, peeled and crushed
Sugar	1 tsp
Water	3–4 litres
Salt	to taste

Chilli sauce

Chicken stock	3 Tbsp
Red chillies	5–6, seeded and sliced
Minced ginger	1 tsp
Garlic	2–3, peeled and minced
Sugar	1 tsp or more to taste
Sesame seed oil	1 tsp
Lime juice	to taste

Method

- To make chicken stock, combine all relevant ingredients in a pot. Boil for 2–3 hours. Ensure that there is at least 3 l liquid at all times. Top up with hot water if liquid reduces too much.

- Preferably done the night before cooking day, refrigerate or freeze cooled stock. Remove solidified fat on top with a spoon. Use as required.

- To make chilli sauce, combine all relevant ingredients and refrigerate.

- Cook rice with sufficient stock instead of water. When done, make rice balls as shown below. Rice has to be hot when you are doing this.

- Bring remaining stock to the boil. Adjust to taste with more salt if desired.

- When liquid is boiling over high heat, add chicken pieces. Leave to boil for about 4–5 minutes. Remove from heat. Drain and slice chicken pieces. Reserve liquid to serve as soup.

- To serve, arrange desired quantities of chicken slices, rice balls, and veggies on individual plates. You may eat bean sprouts raw or blanched in soup. Serve with chilli sauce and soup.

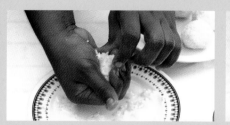 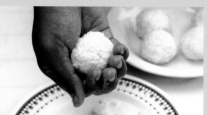

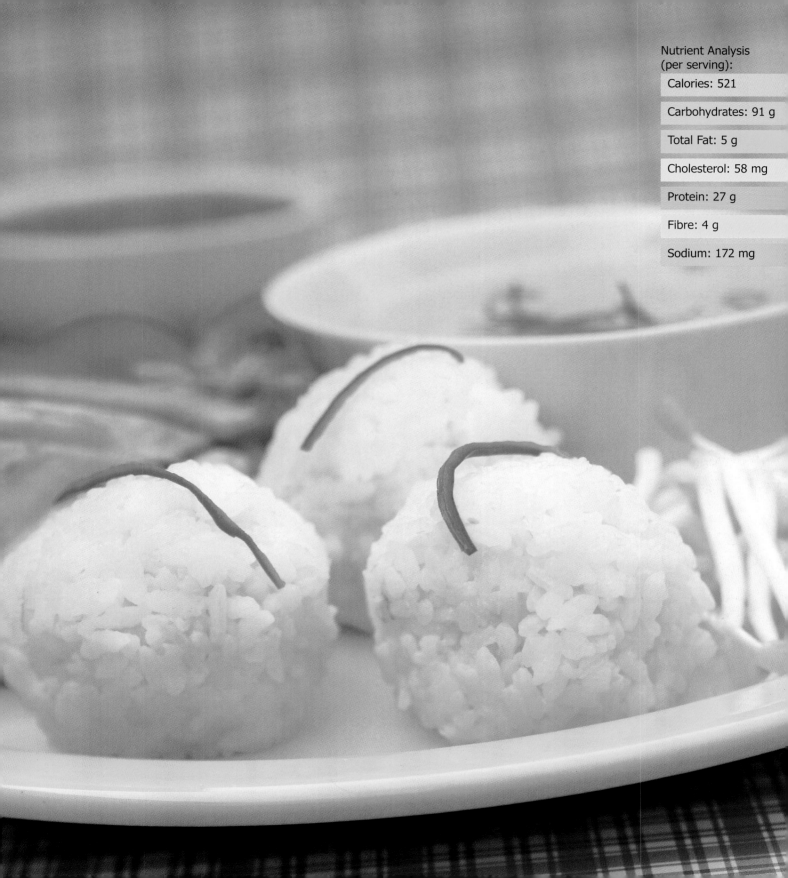

Nutrient Analysis
(per serving):

Calories: 521

Carbohydrates: 91 g

Total Fat: 5 g

Cholesterol: 58 mg

Protein: 27 g

Fibre: 4 g

Sodium: 172 mg

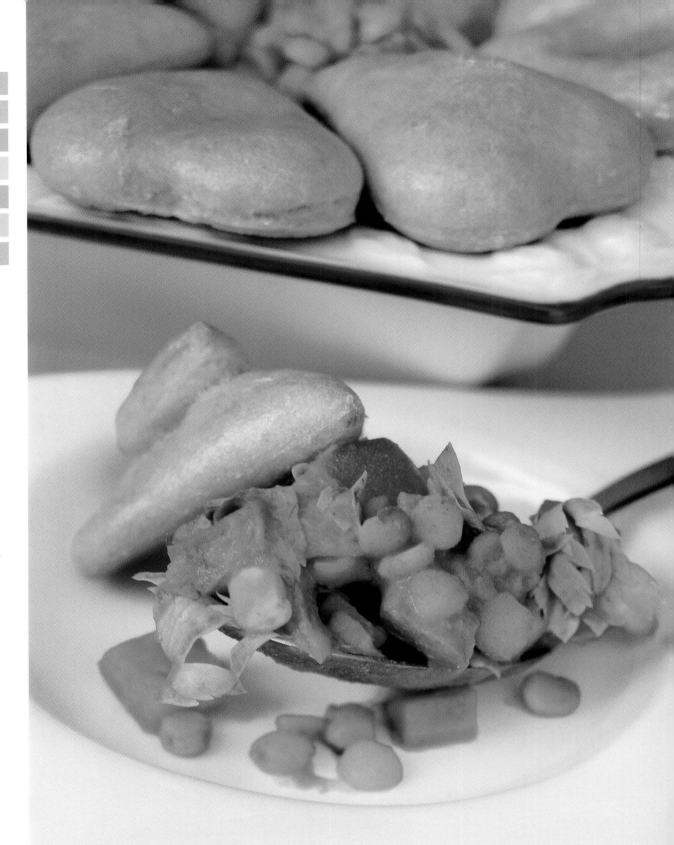

Nutrient Analysis
(per serving):

Calories: 488

Carbohydrates: 76 g

Total Fat: 9 g

Cholesterol: 257 mg

Protein: 32 g

Fibre: 25 g

Sodium: 727 mg

LENTILPIE

Nick's culinary jottings: The first time I ate lentil pie was when I lived in Australia. For some reason, I never liked lentils as a kid but somehow, lentil pie tickled my fancy later in life. I had that one and became totally hooked on them ever since. The degree of spiciness in this recipe is really up to you.

Preparation time : 30 minutes
Cooking time : 45 minutes
Serves 4

Method

- To make crust, first mix flour, salt and baking powder together. Add mustard sauce, apply spray oil and mix well. Set aside.

- Mix egg with rice or soy milk, then add a little at a time to flour mixture to bind into dough. When done, refrigerate.

- Bring stock to the boil in a pot. Add lentils and leave to boil a while. Add onion and curry leaves. Allow to boil until lentils are a little soft.

- Add carrot, celery, cauliflower and curry powder. Leave to boil some more. Add tomatoes and salt and pepper to taste. Simmer until liquid is slightly thick.

- Transfer lentil filling into a heatproof (flameproof) bowl.

- Roll out dough, then cut with cookie cutters of your choice. Arrange dough pieces on top of filling.

- Put pie into oven preheated to 180°C (350°F). Bake until crust is golden brown. Serve warm.

Ingredients

Wholemeal (wholewheat) flour	180 g
Salt	1/2 tsp
Baking powder	1 tsp
Mustard sauce	1 tsp
Spray oil	3 squirts
Egg	1, beaten
Rice or soy milk	180 ml
Stock	500 ml
Lentils	200 g, soaked and drained at least twice
Onion	1, large, peeled and coarsely chopped
Curry leaves	quantity as desired
Carrot	1, medium-size, peeled if desired and cubed
Celery	120 g
Cauliflower	1/2 a head, cut into florets
Curry powder	1 Tbsp
Tomatoes	2, coarsely chopped
Salt and black pepper	to taste

'TEMPERED' DHAL

Nick's culinary jottings: I love to eat this dhal just the way it is with no rice or chapati or naan. Well, frankly speaking, the one I always eat is the not so healthy one with all the oil, but this oil-free version is a good and refreshing change. Tempering this dhal gently brings out the natural flavours of the dhal used. The difference is that we will not be using any oil to temper the ingredients.

Preparation time : 20 minutes (not including soaking of dhal)
Cooking time : 40 minutes
Serves 4

Ingredients

Stock	1 litre
Mung dhal	240 g, replaceable with yellow lentils
Pounded fresh turmeric (*kunyit*)	¹/₂ tsp
Onions	2, large, peeled and coarsely chopped
Ginger	30 g, peeled and minced
Garlic	3 cloves, peeled and minced
Cumin seeds	1 Tbsp, toasted in a dry pan until fragrant and roughly pounded
Mustard seeds	1 Tbsp, toasted in a dry pan until fragrant and roughly pounded
Tomatoes	2, large, roughly chopped
Green chillies	3, seeded and thickly sliced
Carrot	1, grated
Chilli flakes	1 tsp
Salt and pepper	to taste
Lemon juice	to taste
Coriander (cilantro) leaves (optional)	60 g, roughly chopped

Method

- Bring 750 ml of stock to the boil. Add dhal and turmeric and leave to simmer.

- In another pot, sauté onions over low heat with a little stock until fragrant. Add ginger and garlic. Continue to sauté over low heat until fragrant.

- Add cumin and mustard seeds. Add more stock to prevent burning. Add tomatoes, chillies and carrot and leave to cook. When done, combine with boiling dhal.

- To combined ingredients, add chilli flakes and salt and pepper to taste. Then, add sufficient lemon juice to give a slight zing.

- Boil over high heat for about 2–3 minutes, then remove from heat.

- Garnish with coriander leaves and serve hot.

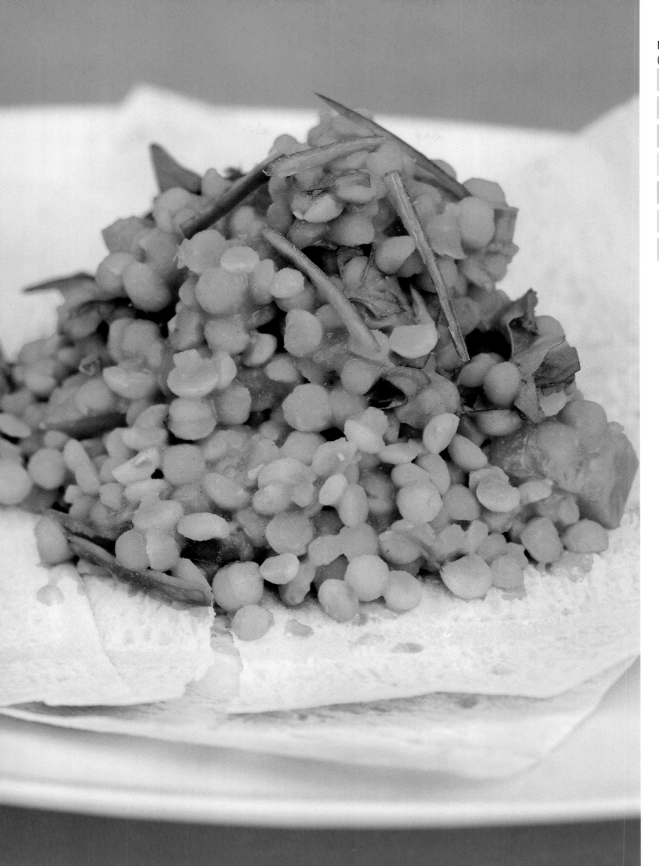

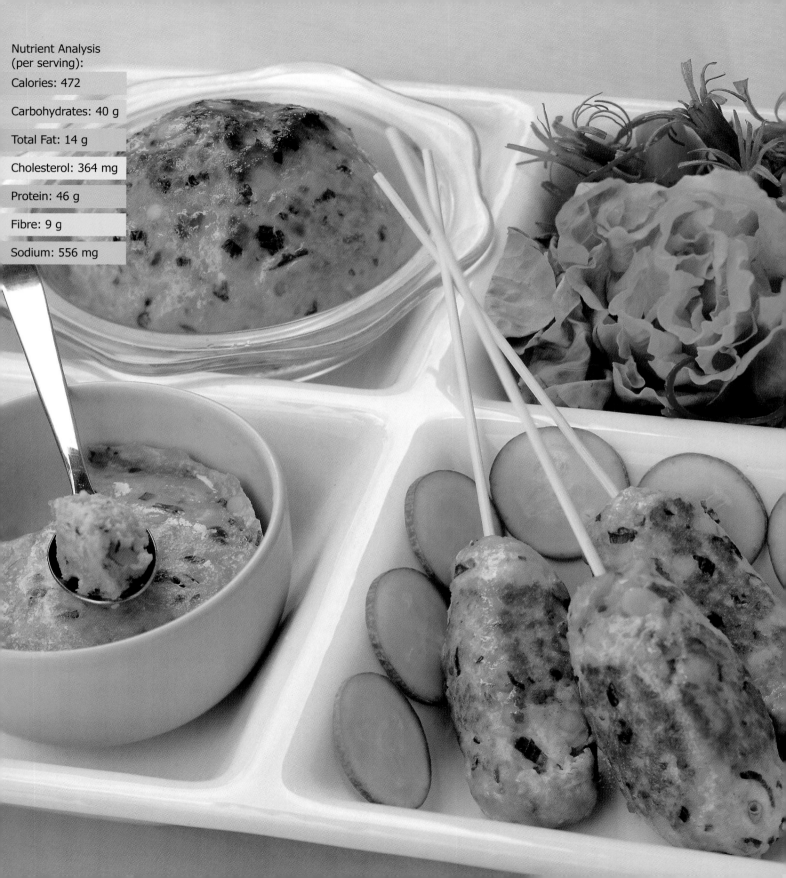

Nutrient Analysis
(per serving):

Calories: 472

Carbohydrates: 40 g

Total Fat: 14 g

Cholesterol: 364 mg

Protein: 46 g

Fibre: 9 g

Sodium: 556 mg

MUNGDHALANDCHICKENKEBABS

Nick's culinary jottings: While this is meant to be a kebab, I changed it a little as one can get lazy sometimes, you know. I usually bake it in the oven in a big casserole dish and once or twice, I have actually steamed it. You know, Indian with a bit of Chinese style. The results, nevertheless, are just as good either way! So you can kebab it, you can bake it or you can steam it. Just try them all, okay? Consider it a typical three-in-one!

Preparation time	: 20 minutes
Cooking time	: 30 minutes
Serves 4	

Method

- Combine all ingredients in a bowl. Leave to marinade for a few hours.

- To kebab it: Form little oval shapes from combined ingredients. Heat a dry pan, then spray on oil when hot. Cook kebabs until done.

- To bake it: Preheat oven to 180°C (350°F). Transfer combined ingredients to a heatproof (flameproof) bowl. Cover and bake until done. It should take around 20–30 minutes, depending on thickness.

- To steam it: Transfer combined ingredients to a heatproof (flameproof) bowl. Steam over high heat for between 13 and 20 minutes.

- Serve any way you like it. Serve with rice, with salad, or even in a sandwich.

Ingredients

Chicken thigh fillets	500 g, minced
Mung dhal	80 g, soaked, boiled until done and drained
Spring onion (scallion)	100 g, finely cut
Low-fat yoghurt	225 g
Green peppercorns	about 20, soaked in salted water, drained, then lightly crushed once or twice with a pestle
Ground ginger	1 tsp
Ground cardamom	1 tsp
Fennel seeds	1¹/₂ tsp, toasted in a dry pan
Rock salt	1 pinch
Fresh breadcrumbs	100 g
Egg	1, large, lightly beaten

Nicholas

It's bad for me to say this... but I am simply not a fan of noodles. I prefer all my local-style noodle dishes to be prepared with pasta instead because I feel the taste is so much better. It's a preference, I guess. Also, having lived overseas could have helped formed my habit as pasta was more readily available and also much cheaper than Chinese noodles.

You should try it, you know and taste the difference in flavours. I also prefer pasta to other carbohydrates because it never leaves me feeling gluggy and heavy after a meal.

Indra

Like rice, noodles and pasta are great sources of complex carbohydrates. A merit of complex carbohydrates is that it releases energy for your body in a slow and steady stream, so it keeps you going for much longer.

The beauty of noodle and pasta dishes is that they are usually complete one-dish meals, making them excellent alternatives for the busy, health-conscious person to keep nutritionally balanced without spending a lot of time. With meat and vegetables added, these noodle and pasta recipes cover the major food groups, so there's no need for you to cook four different dishes. The convenience factor here definitely gets my thumbs up.

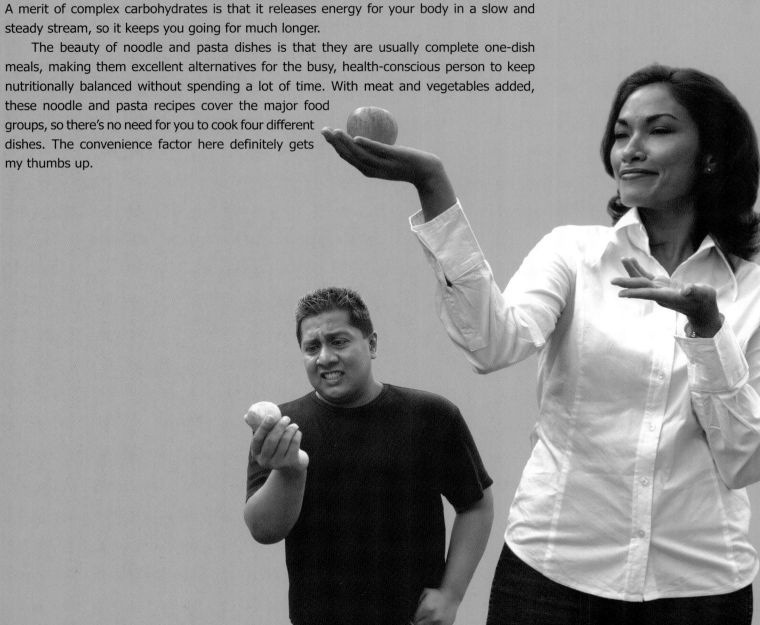

NOODLES AND PASTA

HOKKIEN-STYLE NOODLES

Nick's culinary jottings: This noodle dish has been, without doubt, my utmost favourite since I was a kid. Cooking it with spaghetti came about simply because yellow noodles were quite scarce when I lived overseas, and when I did find them, I couldn't buy them by weight and always wound up having to buy too much. Spaghetti was the cheapest alternative at that time and I have since come to always cook the dish with pasta after that. The result, I feel, is so much better with spaghetti.

Preparation time : 20 minutes
Cooking time : 20 minutes (not including boiling of pasta)
Serves 4

Ingredients

Chicken fillet	100 g, cut into strips
Chicken liver (optional)	100 g, sliced
Chicken gizzard (optional)	100 g, boiled and sliced
Light soy sauce	to taste
Pepper	to taste
Sugar	to taste
Medium–large prawns (shrimps)	100 g, peeled and deveined
Squid tubes	100 g, sliced
Crabmeat	100 g
Dark soy sauce	5–6 Tbsp
Fish sauce	1 Tbsp
Stock	375 ml
Garlic	4 cloves, peeled and minced
Spray oil	2 squirts
Salt	to taste
Chinese flowering cabbage (*choy sum* or *sawi*)	10 stalks, leaves and stems separated, then cut into bite-size lengths
Spaghetti	300 g, boiled until al dente and drained
Cabbage leaves	5–6, sliced
Corn flour (cornstarch)	1 Tbsp, mixed with a little water to make thickener

Method

- In a bowl, combine chicken meat, liver and gizzard if used. Season with light soy sauce, pepper and sugar to taste. Set aside. Repeat with all seafood combined and set aside.

- In a third bowl, combine dark soy sauce and fish sauce. Add pepper and sugar to taste. Set aside.

- Bring 2–3 Tbsp stock to the boil in a saucepan. Add garlic and apply spray oil. Stir continuously until slightly fragrant.

- Add remaining stock. Bring to another boil. Add seasoned chicken, then seafood. Simmer for about 3 minutes.

- Add combined sauces. Add more dark soy sauce if you prefer a dish darker in colour. Adjust to taste with more pepper and salt if desired.

- Add flowering cabbage stems, then leaves. Leave to cook for 2 minutes. Add spaghetti and cabbage. Bring to the boil over high heat.

- Stir in corn flour mixture. When liquid thickens, remove from heat and serve.

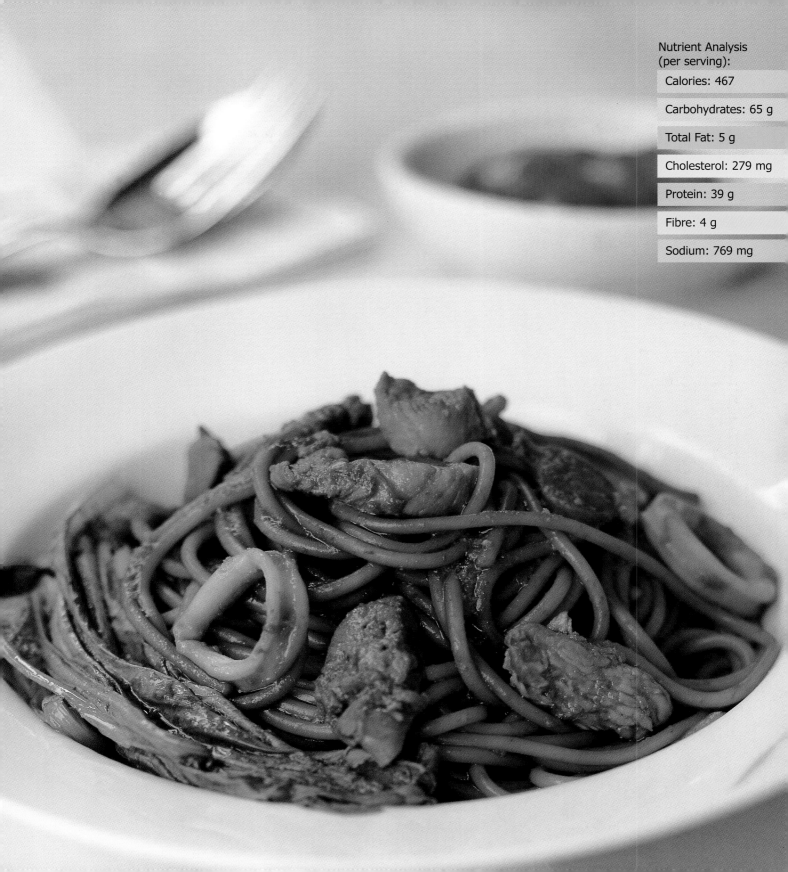

Nutrient Analysis
(per serving):

Calories: 467

Carbohydrates: 65 g

Total Fat: 5 g

Cholesterol: 279 mg

Protein: 39 g

Fibre: 4 g

Sodium: 769 mg

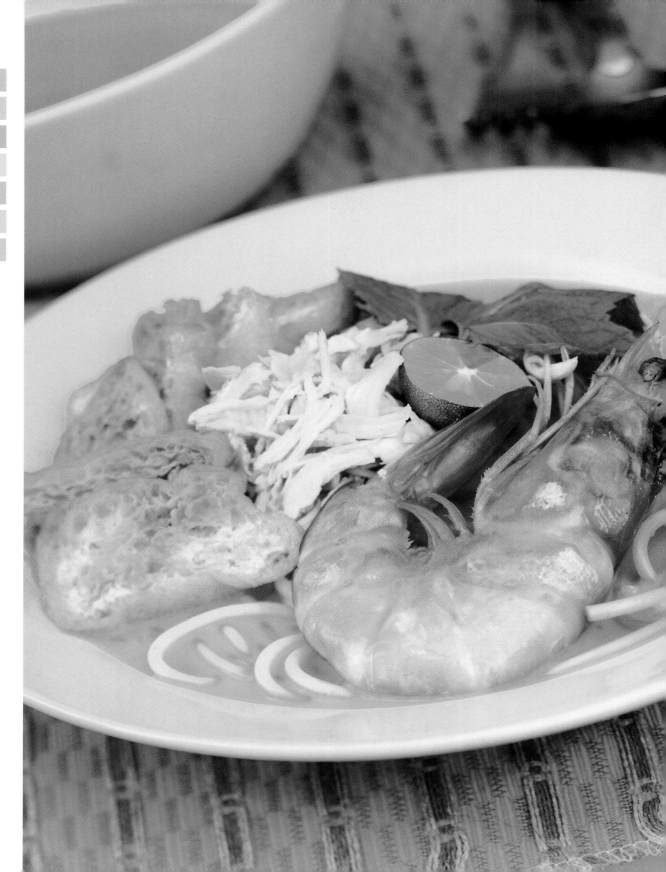

Nutrient Analysis
(per serving):

Calories: 275 g

Carbohydrates: 33 g

Total Fat: 6 g

Cholesterol: 54 mg

Protein: 27 g

Fibre: 3 g

Sodium: 544 mg

CURRYLAKSA

Preparation time : 30 minutes (does not include stock-boiling)
Cooking time : 30 minutes
Serves 6

Nick's culinary jottings: One can never get enough of curry *laksa*, well, at least not my family. We can eat and eat and eat like it's going out of style only to regret later when we start feeling the ill effects of the rich coconut milk used. For the last ten years, I have never ever bought *laksa* from a shop simply because my mother made the nicest *laksa* and I learnt how to prepare it from her.

Method

- Combine chicken bones, anchovies and water in a pot. Boil for a few hours. Skim off fat.

- If time allows, freeze cooled stock and remove all solidified fat with a spoon.

- Strain stock before use.

- Heat a dry pan. Add ground ingredients and a little stock. Stir until fragrant. Apply spray oil. Add sugar and salt to taste. Stir until tiny bits of oil appear on the top.

- Add remaining stock and bring to the boil. Add all milk and simmer; do not over-boil.

- Serve with noodles and complementary ingredients of your choice.

♗ Note: Vietnamese mint leaves are also known as polygonum leaves.

♗ Indra's note: Because dried anchovies are high in sodium, rinsing them several times helps to remove excess salt, while removing the heads of the anchovies helps to cut down the amount of cholesterol.

Ingredients

Chicken bones	500 g
Dried anchovies	100 g, heads removed, rinsed several times and drained
Water	5 litres
Spray oil	2 squirts
Sugar	1 Tbsp
Salt	to taste
Soy milk	750 ml
Rice milk	250 ml

Ingredients to be ground (processed)

Dried chillies	20–30, soaked and drained
Onions	5–6, large, peeled
Garlic	10 cloves, peeled
Candlenuts (*buah keras*)	12
Fresh turmeric (*kunyit*)	1 small knob, peeled
Galangal (*lengkuas*)	4-cm knob, peeled
Lemon grass (*serai*)	8 stalks
Dried prawns (shrimps) (*ha mai*)	4 Tbsp
Dried prawn (shrimp) paste (*belacan*)	1½ Tbsp
Torch ginger bud (*bunga kantan*)	1 stalk

Complementary ingredients

Bean curd puffs (*tau pok*)	10, sliced into bite-size pieces
Shredded chicken meat	quantity as desired
Prawns (shrimps)	quantity as desired
Bean sprouts	quantity as desired
Vietnamese mint (*daun kesum*)	a few sprigs
Sliced red chillies	quantity as desired
Halved kalamansi limes	quantity as desired

THAISEAFOODNOODLESALAD

Nick's culinary jottings: This cold salad dish was concocted when my friend Salmah Khalid bought glass noodles (*fun see*) instead of rice vermicelli (*mai fun*) one day. She bought too much of it too and so I had to think of something as I was brought up not to waste any food. So, this one's for you Salmah. Eaten on a hot summer's day or a hot Malaysian afternoon, it is light and refreshing and won't make you feel too full.

Preparation time : 15 minutes
Cooking time : 10 minutes
Serves 4

Ingredients

Squid tubes	3, sliced
Large prawns (shrimps)	200 g, peeled and deveined
Fish fillet	200 g, cut into bite-size pieces
Glass noodles (*fun see*)	200 g, boiled until cooked, drained and refrigerated
Chopped spring onions (scallions)	

Sauce

Sweet chilli sauce	5 Tbsp
Ground black pepper	1 tsp
Garlic	1 clove, peeled and minced
Sesame seed oil	1 tsp
Light soy sauce	1 Tbsp
Lemon juice	to taste
Sugar	to taste

Method

- Combine sauce ingredients in a small pot. Bring to the boil over low heat.

- Add all seafood and stir until cooked. This should take about 3–4 minutes.

- When done, pour liquid over glass noodles and mix well. Reserve seafood pieces separately.

- Refrigerate noodles and seafood. Serve cold. Garnish with chopped spring onions if desired.

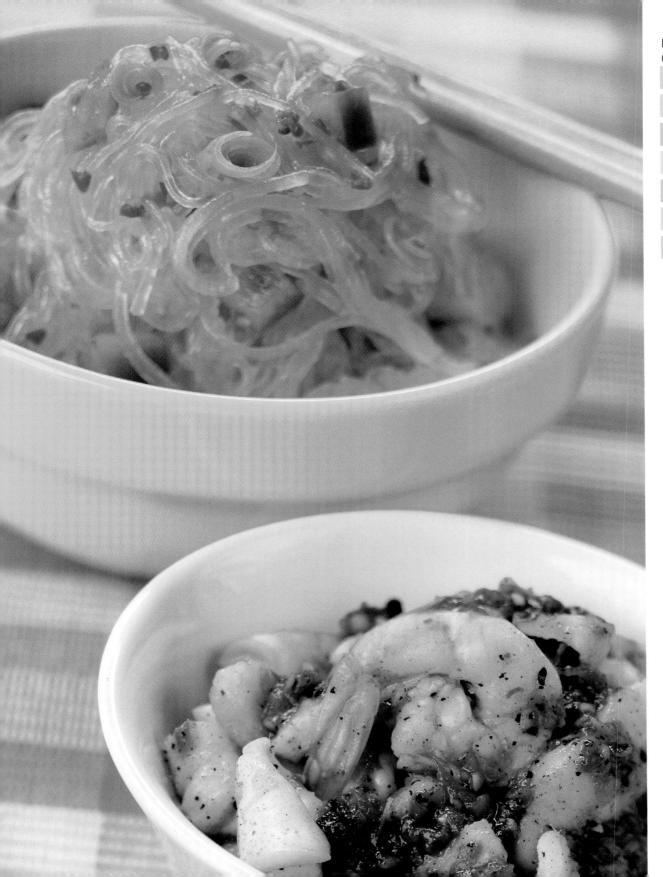

Nutrient Analysis
(per serving):

Calories: 285

Carbohydrates: 50 g

Total Fat: 2 g

Cholesterol: 134 mg

Protein: 17 g

Fibre: 1 g

Sodium: 409 mg

Nutrient Analysis
(per serving):

Calories: 725

Carbohydrates: 128 g

Total Fat: 18 g

Cholesterol: 131 mg

Protein: 42 g

Fibre: 14 g

Sodium: 855 mg

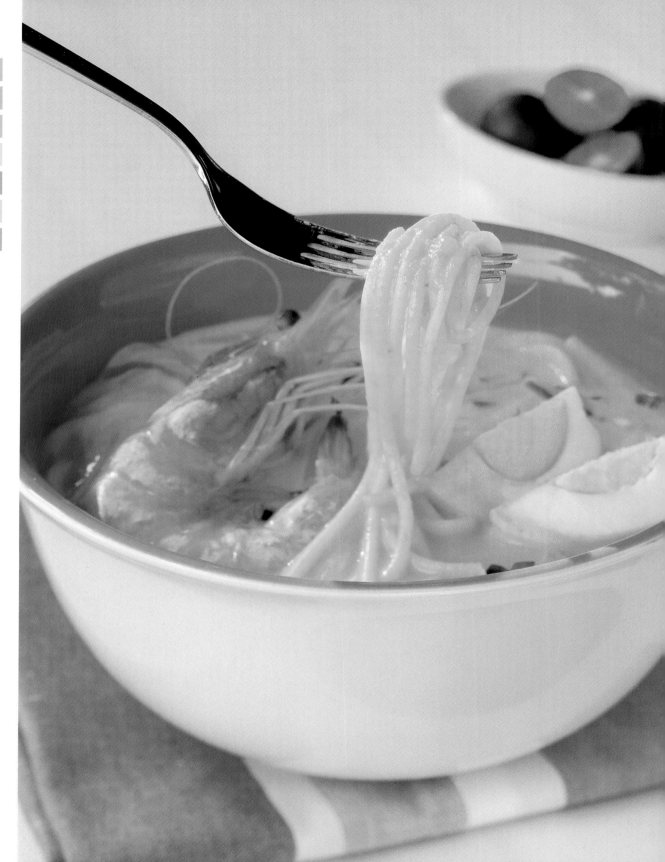

MEEREBUS

Nick's culinary jottings: This Malaysian favourite has been around for ages, and this recipe is a culmination of several recipes that I have used in the past with excellent results. I use spaghetti instead of the usual yellow noodles simply because I do not like the additives and the funny aftertaste yellow noodles sometimes have. Use prawn shells to make the stock but if you have a guest with an allergy, then use chicken stock.

Preparation time : 30 minutes
Cooking time : 60 minutes
Serves 6

Method

- Grind (process) onions, lemon grass, galangal, chillies, garlic, dried prawns and dried prawn paste together.

- In a large pot, spray on oil and sauté ground ingredients. Add a little stock to infuse flavours more effectively.

- Add remaining stock. Leave to boil until liquid is almost halved.

- Add sugar and salt to taste. Leave to boil for a few minutes more. Add sweet potato to thicken.

- To serve, portion spaghetti into individual serving bowls. Ladle hot gravy over.

- Arrange complementary ingredients buffet style at the table for family or guests to self-select and enjoy.

Ingredients

Onions	3, large, peeled
Lemon grass (*serai*)	6 stalks
Young galangal (*lengkuas*)	100 g, peeled
Red chillies	5–6 or more to taste
Garlic	3–4 cloves, peeled
Dried prawns (shrimps) (*ha mai*)	150 g, toasted in a dry pan
Dried prawn (shrimp) paste (*belacan*)	2 tsp
Spray oil	3–4 squirts
Stock	4 litres
Sugar	1 Tbsp
Salt	to taste
Orange-fleshed sweet potato	about 1 kg, peeled, boiled and finely mashed
Spaghetti	500 g, boiled until al dente and drained

Complementary ingredients

Hard boiled eggs	3, shelled and quartered
Bean sprouts	about 300 g, may be blanched or left raw
Chinese celery leaves	a few sprigs, roughly chopped
Kalamansi limes	5–6 or more to taste, halved
Large prawns (shrimps)	quantity as desired
Spring onions (scallions)	quantity as desired, chopped
Bird's eye chillies (*cili padi*)	quantity as desired, sliced

AUSH

Nick's culinary jottings: The first time I ate this noodle dish, I had a coating of oil left on my lips. It was good nevertheless and well worth the time spent to make it. It is also a one-pot wonder, of course, and rather healthy despite the oil. In Afghanistan, from which this recipe originates, *aush* is eaten during winter which explains its richness. This wholesome dish is full of proteins and carbohydrates and can be served at any meal.

Preparation time	: 60 minutes
Cooking time	: 60 minutes
Serves 6	

Ingredients

Spinach	1 kg, leaves and stems separated
Kidney beans	130 g, soaked for a few hours
Yellow lentils	160 g, soaked for a few hours
Salt and pepper	to taste
Aush noodles*	1 recipe, boiled in salted water until al dente and drained
Lamb sauce*	1 recipe
Yoghurt dressing*	1 recipe

Method

- Boil spinach in some water until cooked. Drain and leave to cool. Chop up cooled spinach.
- Separately boil kidney beans and lentils in salted water until done, then drain.
- Mix spinach, beans and lentils together. Add salt and pepper to taste. Set aside.
- Put cooked noodles into a large heatproof (flameproof) bowl. Ladle on lamb sauce. Add spinach mixture over sauce and yoghurt dressing on top.
- If preferred, bake in an oven preheated to 220°C (440°F) until lightly golden. Serve hot. Alternatively, eat it without baking.

*(refer to p. 92–93)

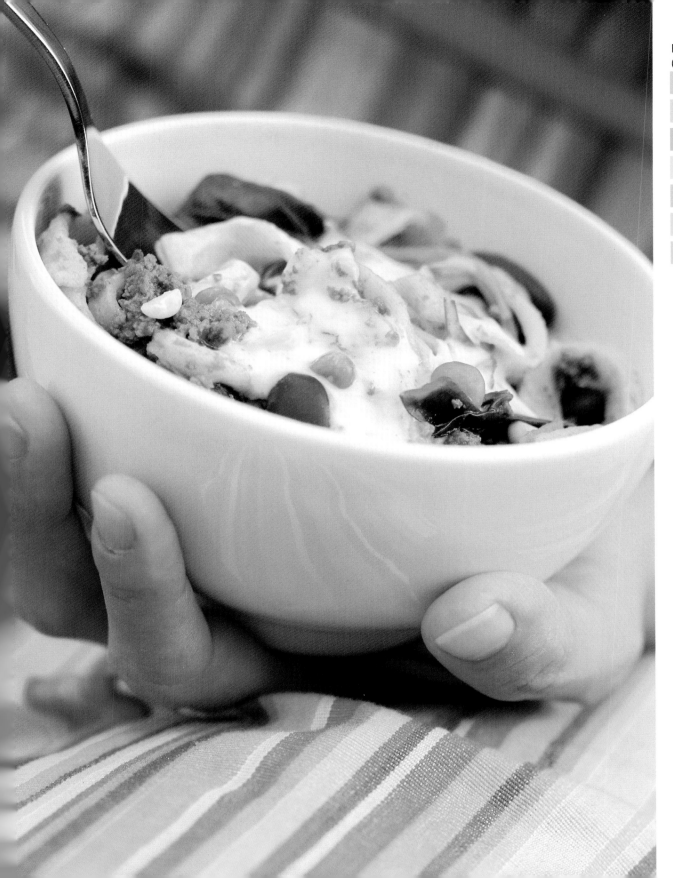

Nutrient Analysis
(per serving):

Calories: 686

Carbohydrates: 86 g

Total Fat: 21 g

Cholesterol: 91 mg

Protein: 41 g

Fibre: 16 g

Sodium: 453 mg

AUSH

Aush noodles

Bread flour	375 g and a little more to knead
Ground black pepper	1 Tbsp
Salt	to taste
Egg	1, lightly beaten
Cold water	125 ml

Method

- In a bowl, combine flour, pepper and salt. Mix well, then shape into a well. Add egg in the centre and start kneading.

- Add water little by little, kneading continuously. Depending on the flour and the humidity of the day, you sometimes do not need all of the water and at other times need more.

- When done, cover bowl with cling film (plastic wrap). Set aside for about 30 minutes.

- On a floured board, roll out dough to a thin rectangle. Roll rectangle up Swiss-roll style, then slice from short end. It is really up to you how thick or thin you want the noodles to be.

- When done slicing, open up noodles and leave them for a while to dry out.

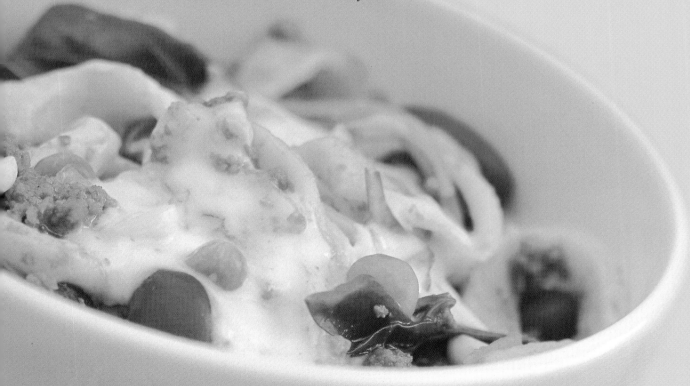

Method

- Combine all dressing ingredients. Refrigerate to improve taste, so flavours can infuse.

Method

- In a pot, sear onions over low heat. As they start to brown, apply spray oil. Sauté over low heat until fragrant.

- Add cumin seeds, then garlic and tomato paste. Stir until fragrant. Add stock and leave to boil for a few minutes.

- Add meat and stir to mix. Simmer until meat is cooked through.

- Mix in powdered ingredients. Adjust to taste with salt and pepper. Simmer over low heat for about 10 minutes. If it is very dry, add more stock.

- Add peas and allow to cook for a few minutes more. Remove from heat.

Yoghurt dressing

Plain low-fat yoghurt	450 g
Fresh mint leaves	30 g, finely chopped
Chilli flakes	1 tsp or more to taste
Coriander (cilantro) leaves	30 g, finely chopped
Lemon juice	to taste

Lamb sauce

Onions	3, large, peeled and cubed
Spray oil	
Cumin seeds	3 tsp
Garlic	2 cloves, peeled and minced
Tomato paste	130 g
Stock	250 ml
Lean minced lamb	500 g
Ground coriander (cilantro)	1½ Tbsp
Curry powder	1 Tbsp or more to taste
Ground cinnamon	1 tsp
Salt and black pepper	to taste
Green peas	100 g

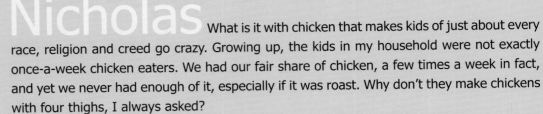

Nicholas

What is it with chicken that makes kids of just about every race, religion and creed go crazy. Growing up, the kids in my household were not exactly once-a-week chicken eaters. We had our fair share of chicken, a few times a week in fact, and yet we never had enough of it, especially if it was roast. Why don't they make chickens with four thighs, I always asked?

Because chicken is a white meat, it is often presumed to be less fatty, but this is certainly not true. Try roasting a chicken with one of those vertical chicken roaster contraptions, where your chicken literally stands in the oven over a bowl, and I am very certain you will be shocked by the amount of oil collected at the end of cooking time. No matter how many times I have done it, the resulting oil never fails to flabbergast me. It's just shocking, so let's see what Indra has to say about all this.

Indra

Yessiree folks, Nicholas is right — chicken meat by itself is very high in protein and relatively low in fat. The fat in chicken is found mainly in or near the skin, so if you want to cut down on the fat content of your chicken dishes, simply remove the skin.

When it comes to cooking the chicken, however, the skin is what gives it that delicious flavour and moistness. A friend of mine, who had to change his dietary habits after undergoing heart bypass surgery, maintains that eating dry chicken breast meat is worse than eating his own shoe! This friend of mine had read in books that chicken breast was the ideal choice for people on a low-fat diet.

The rule of thumb is you can make a roast chicken with the skin on, but do not eat the skin. Also, use a proper grilling rack when cooking so that the oil from the skin drains away from the chicken.

CHICKEN

CHICKEN CURRY

Nick's culinary jottings: Chicken curry to us in Southeast Asia is like chicken broth to those in the West. It is the most commonly cooked curry and yet, no one household can actually emulate the other. This recipe is my mother's minus the coconut milk, of course. Her recipe is a good blend of how the Chinese and the Indians like their curries.

Preparation time : 20 minutes
Cooking time : 40–45 minutes
Serves 4

Ingredients

Chicken thighs and drumsticks	1 kg, skinned and excess fat trimmed
Meat curry powder	3 Tbsp
Salt	1 tsp
Chilli powder	1 tsp
Cinnamon stick	1, about 3 cm
Star anise	2
Cloves	6
Cardamoms	3
Ground coriander (cilantro)	1 Tbsp
Ground cumin	1 Tbsp
Ground sweet cumin	1 tsp
Curry leaves	4 sprigs, stems discarded
Unsweetened soy milk	375 ml
Salt and pepper	to taste

Ingredients to be blended (processed)

Onions	2, large, peeled
Garlic	1 clove, peeled
Ginger	50 g, peeled
Red chillies	3

Method

- Season chicken with 1 Tbsp curry powder, salt and chilli powder. Set aside.

- Combine 500 ml water and blended ingredients in a pot. Simmer for about 10 minutes.

- Add cinnamon stick, star anise, cloves and cardamoms. Simmer for 10 minutes more.

- Except soy milk, salt and pepper, add remaining ingredients. Leave to boil for another 10 minutes or until fragrant. If too dry, add more water. The heat should be low but steady throughout cooking time.

- Add chicken pieces. Simmer for 20–25 minutes, depending on size of chicken pieces. Stir occasionally. Cover pot if desired.

- Finally, add soy milk. Simmer for 10 minutes more.

- Adjust to taste with salt and pepper. Add more curry powder for a spicier dish.

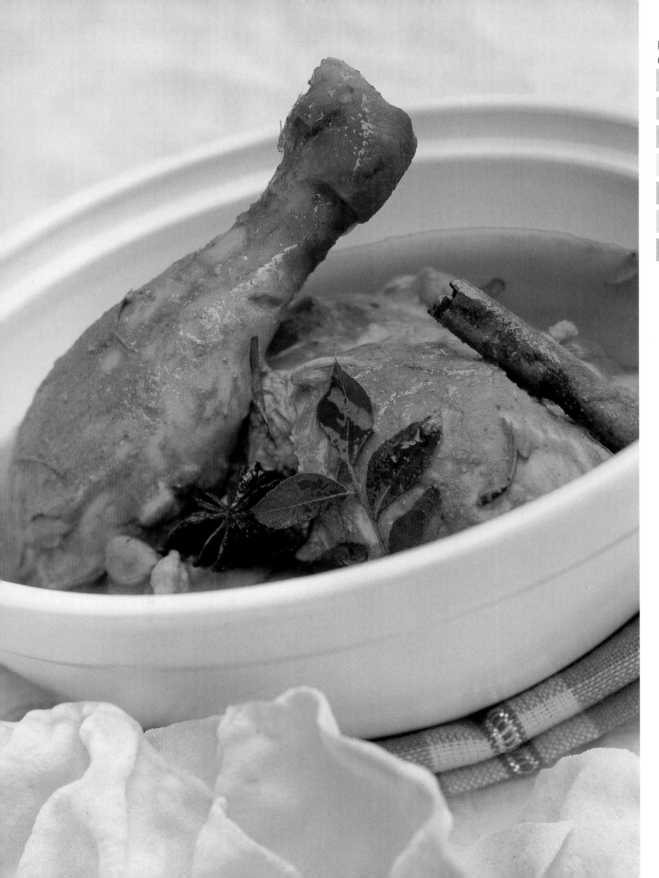

Nutrient Analysis
(per serving):

Calories: 509

Carbohydrates: 19 g

Total Fat: 23 g

Cholesterol: 150 mg

Protein: 51 g

Fibre: 3 g

Sodium: 697 mg

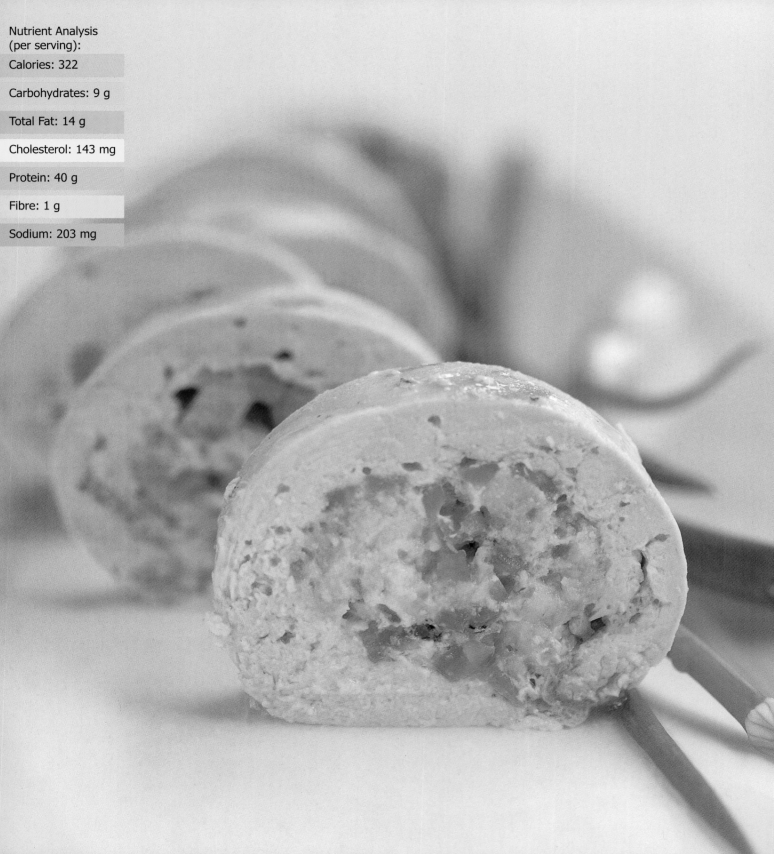

Nutrient Analysis
(per serving):

Calories: 322

Carbohydrates: 9 g

Total Fat: 14 g

Cholesterol: 143 mg

Protein: 40 g

Fibre: 1 g

Sodium: 203 mg

CHICKEN ROULADE WITH SEAFOOD STUFFING

Nick's culinary jottings: This tricky-sounding recipe is actually very easy to make. It is not messy and it does not take much time either. The visual effect of it is simply marvellous, and the combination of flavours makes you want to reach out for more but don't worry, eat and be happy, because it's almost fat free.

Preparation time	: 30–40 minutes
Cooking time	: 10–15 minutes
Serves 4	

Method

- Flatten out chicken breasts with a meat mallet. Season with salt and pepper. Set aside.

- Set up steamer and leave it to boil. Steam stock with chicken bones for a richer soup if desired.

- Spoon sufficient fish paste onto chicken. Roll as you would sushi. Secure with toothpicks (cocktail sticks) as shown below, or tie with cotton string so roll will not undo.

- Add chicken roulade to stock. Steam for about 10 minutes.

- Remove roulade from soup. Remove toothpicks or string. Slice from short end. Arrange slices on a platter. Ladle some soup over to moisten if necessary.

Ingredients

Chicken breasts	4
Salt and pepper	to taste
Stock	250 ml, hot
Chicken bones (optional)	
Fish paste*	1 recipe

Method

- Blend (process) mackerel until paste-like. Transfer to a bowl.

- Season with pepper, sesame seed oil, oyster sauce and fish sauce to taste.

- Mix in carrot, onion, coriander and lemon grass. Add corn flour to bind paste.

*Fish paste

Mackerel fish fillet	250 g
Ground black pepper	1 tsp
Sesame seed oil	1 tsp
Oyster sauce	1 tsp
Fish sauce	to taste
Carrot	1, small, peeled if desired and minced
Onion	1, small, peeled and minced
Coriander (cilantro)	30 g, chopped
Lemon grass (*serai*)	1 stalk, thinly sliced
Corn flour (cornstarch)	1 Tbsp

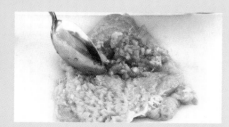
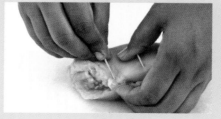

CASHEWNUTCHICKEN

Nick's culinary jottings: This was often the highlight of eating at a Chinese restaurant when we were kids. The fattest part of this recipe was the cashew nuts. Before, however, cashew nut chicken literally meant pieces of chicken with very few cashew nuts. It's much better these days. Roast your own cashew nuts or buy the ones that have been roasted instead of fried. Aside from oil, that's a good way to cut down on sodium too, as most of the prepacked variety have added salt.

Preparation time : 20–30 minutes
Cooking time : 20 minutes
Serves 6

Ingredients

Chicken thigh fillets	500 g, skinned, excess fat trimmed and cut into strips
Ground black pepper	to taste
Sesame seed oil	to taste
Fish sauce	to taste
Sugar	1 tsp or more to taste
Onions	4–5, peeled and each cut into 5–6 wedges
Stock	375 ml
Garlic	3 cloves, peeled and minced
Oyster sauce	3 Tbsp
Black vinegar	1 Tbsp
Dried chillies	5–6, cut into bite-size pieces
Carrot	1, peeled if desired and sliced
Red capsicum (sweet bell pepper)	2, cut to the same size as onion pieces
Green capsicum (sweet bell pepper)	1, cut as above
Yam bean (*bang kuang*)	2, small, peeled and cut into cubes
Corn flour (cornstarch)	1 Tbsp, mixed with a little water to make thickener
Roasted cashew nuts	135 g

Method

- Lightly season chicken with pepper, sesame seed oil, fish sauce, and a pinch of sugar. Set aside.

- Brown onions in a dry pan. Once they start to leave brown marks on pan's surface, pour in stock and add garlic.

- Add oyster sauce, vinegar and 1 tsp sugar, as well as pepper and fish sauce to taste. Leave to simmer for 2–3 minutes. Add dried chillies. Simmer for 1–2 minutes more.

- Add carrot and simmer for 1 minute, then capsicums and yam bean. Stir through.

- Add chicken. Leave to boil over high heat for 4–5 minutes, stirring continuously.

- Add corn flour mixture. When liquid thickens, sprinkle on some cashew nuts, stir and dish out.

- Sprinkle on more cashew nuts if desired. Serve with rice.

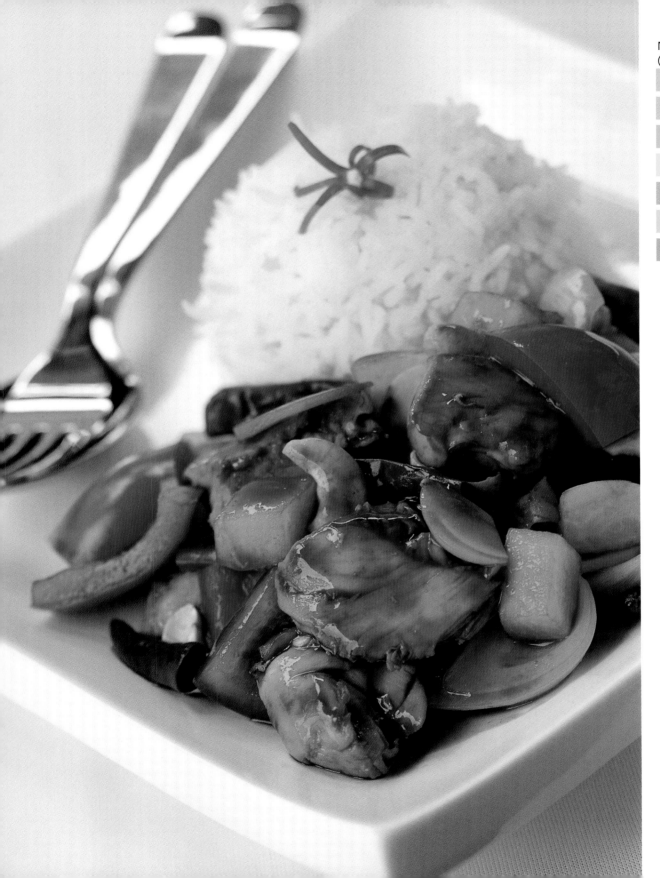

Nutrient Analysis
(per serving):

Calories: 395

Carbohydrates: 24 g

Total Fat: 25 g

Cholesterol: 82 mg

Protein: 28 g

Fibre: 3 g

Sodium: 364 mg

Nutrient Analysis
(per serving):

Calories: 345

Carbohydrates: 12 g

Total Fat: 22 g

Cholesterol: 126 mg

Protein: 25 g

Fibre: 1 g

Sodium: 270 mg

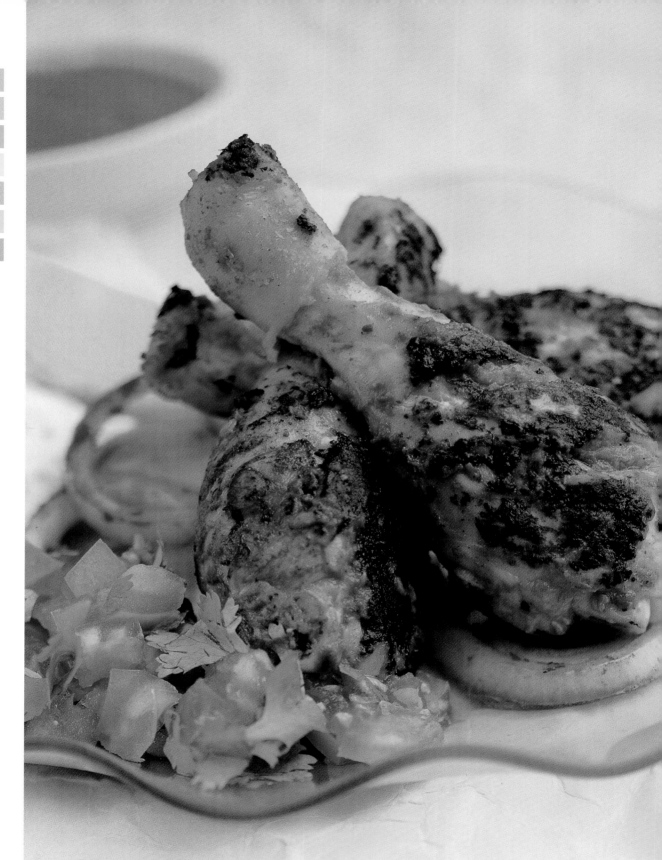

CHICKEN TIKKA

Nick's culinary jottings: This *tikka* recipe is cooked partly in a nonstick pan and then cooked *dum* method in an oven on low until you need to serve it. *Dum* is a method of cooking that involves cooking food in its own steam in a sealed environment.

Preparation time : 15 minutes
Cooking time : 20–30 minutes
Serves 4

Method

- Combine all marinade ingredients in a large bowl. Add chicken and leave to marinate for at least 8 hours, or preferably overnight.

- Apply spray oil onto nonstick pan. Lightly sear chicken pieces, then leave for 2–3 minutes. Transfer to a tray lined with tin foil. Pour marinade on top. Cover with more foil.

- Preheat oven to 100°C (212°F). Bake chicken for at least 45 minutes. Keep warm in oven until you are about to serve.

- Sprinkle on desired amounts of lemon juice and *chaat masala* before serving.

Note: *Chaat masala*, like *garam masala,* is an Indian spice mixture that is sold ready-mixed in most supermarkets.

Ingredients

Chicken thighs or thigh fillets	500 g
Spray oil	1 squirt
Lemon juice	to taste
Chaat masala	to taste

Marinade

Grated ginger	2 Tbsp
Grated garlic	2 Tbsp
Ground nutmeg	1 tsp
Mace	1 tsp
Garam masala	1 Tbsp
Chilli powder	1 Tbsp
Tomato paste	3 Tbsp
Coriander (cilantro) seeds	1 Tbsp, roughly ground
Plain low-fat yogurt	225 g
Pepper	1 tsp
Salt	to taste

FRENCHBAGUETTEWITHSPICY CHICKENSTUFFING

Nick's culinary jottings: This is one recipe that is not only easy but also a conversation piece. Serve it on one of those days when friends are over to watch a DVD or just for a chat.

Preparation time : 15 minutes
Cooking time : 30 minutes
Serves 6

Ingredients

French baguette	1, cut into thirds
Minced chicken	500 g
Soy milk	125 ml
Onion	1, peeled and minced
Garlic	2 cloves, peeled and minced
Cumin	1 tsp
Ground coriander (cilantro)	1 tsp
Fennel seeds	1 tsp, toasted in a dry pan
Curry powder	1 Tbsp
Fresh coriander (cilantro) leaves	30 g, roughly chopped
Salt	to taste
Egg	1

Method

- Without breaking skin, remove as much as possible white, fluffy parts of baguette pieces.

- In a pan, sear chicken. Add soy milk and cook for about 3 minutes. Except egg, add remaining ingredients. Leave to simmer for a few minutes more or until done.

- Remove from heat and leave to cool for a few minutes. Break egg into filling and mix well.

- Preheat oven to 170°C (340°F).

- Stuff filling into baguette shells until taut. Wrap each piece in tin foil, then place on baking tray.

- Bake for 15–20 minutes. Just before removing from oven, tear away foil on top and let exposed parts brown a little more.

- Slice rolls with a very sharp knife, but not too thin or pieces will fall apart. Serve immediately.

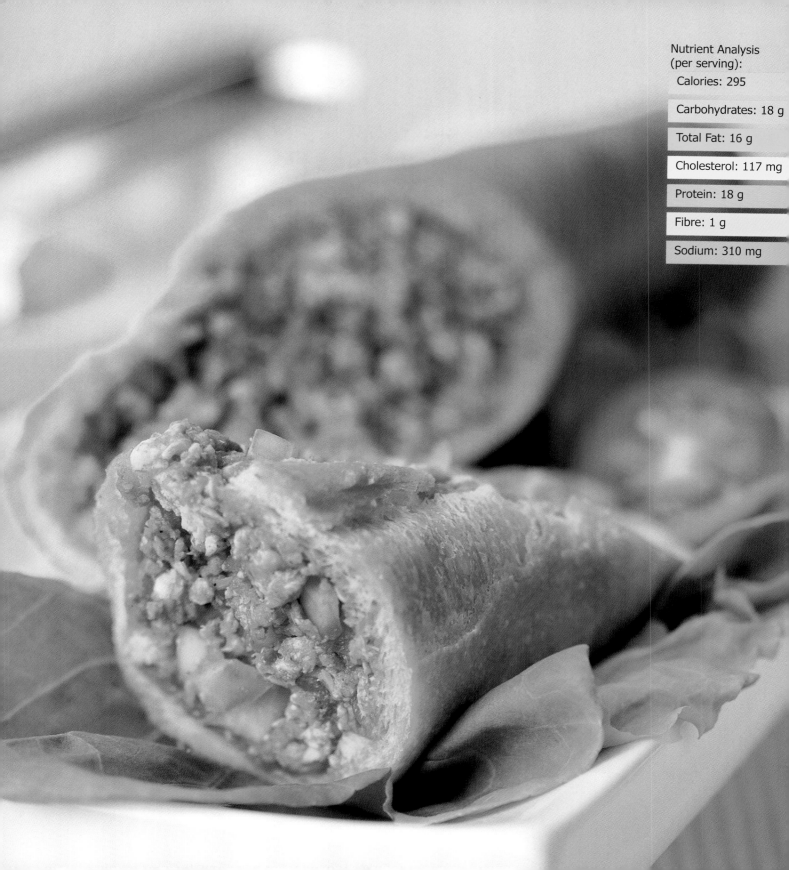

Nutrient Analysis
(per serving):
Calories: 295

Carbohydrates: 18 g

Total Fat: 16 g

Cholesterol: 117 mg

Protein: 18 g

Fibre: 1 g

Sodium: 310 mg

Nutrient Analysis
(per serving):

Calories: 192

Carbohydrates: 14 g

Total Fat: 8 g

Cholesterol: 210 mg

Protein: 16 g

Fibre: 1 g

Sodium: 258 mg

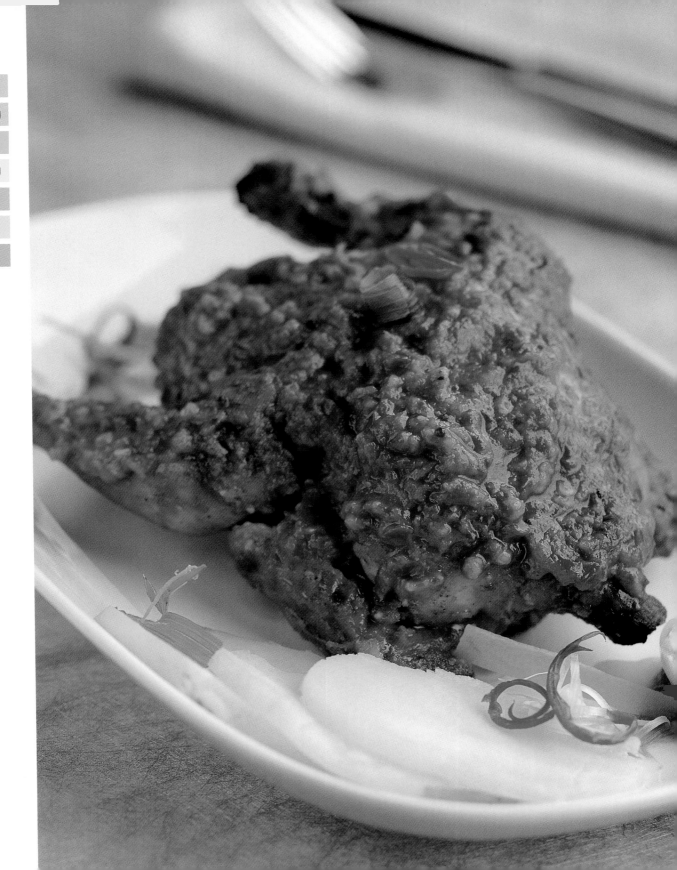

AYAM GOLEK

Nick's culinary jottings: This recipe is an old-fashioned, Malay-style roast. In Malay villages a long time ago, the dish was cooked using charcoal and coconut husks. The traditional way also meant a richly fat-laden roast chicken, although free range, which I have to say is to die for. These days, however, we have to watch what we are eating and cook this the healthy way. I have chosen to leave the skin on because there is nothing worse than dry roast chicken in my books, but you may wish to take off the skin after the chicken is cooked.

Preparation time : 30 minutes
Cooking time : 60 minutes
Serves 5

Method

- Season chicken with a little salt and pepper. Set aside.
- Combine pounded and blended ingredients in a pot. Add sugar and water. Bring to the boil. Simmer until liquid is halved and fragrant.
- Season to taste with salt. Add soy milk. Leave to boil for 10 minutes or until liquid is halved again.
- Combine all stuffing ingredients in a bowl. Add two ladlefuls of reduced liquid and ingredients. Mix well.
- Stuff chicken and stitch up so stuffing will not fall out.
- Bake chicken in oven preheated to 180°C (350°F) for about 1 hour. Baste with remaining liquid every 20 minutes to keep flesh moist. When done, serve with hot rice or some salad.

Ingredients

Chicken	1, head, neck and feet removed and cleaned
Salt and pepper	to taste
Sugar	1 tsp
Water	500 ml
Soy milk	250 ml

Ingredients to be coarsely pounded

Cinnamon stick	1, 3–4 cm
Cloves	3
Black peppercorns	10
Ground coriander (cilantro)	1 Tbsp
Fennel seeds	1 tsp
Cumin	1 tsp

Ingredients to be blended (processed)

Onion	1, large, peeled and chopped
Lemon grass (*serai*)	1 stalk
Red chillies	3
Garlic	3–4 cloves, peeled
Ginger	2-cm knob, peeled
Dried prawn (shrimp) paste (*belacan*)	1 Tbsp

Stuffing

Potatoes	150 g, boiled and cubed
Quail's eggs	10, hard boiled and shelled
Vietnamese mint leaves (*daun kesum*)	1 stalk, thinly sliced
Chicken livers	2, boiled and mashed

Nicholas

Cooking with ostrich is a favourite of mine simply because no one would have eaten it a few years ago. Ostrich meat is one of the most fat-free meats around and is also tender, flavoursome and, most importantly, easy to cook.

Until I tried ostrich for the first time, I never knew a meat could taste so nice. It had the consistency of good beef and chicken. The meat was red too and I had it with a black pepper sauce. From then on, the whole family came to love ostrich.

I do feel a tinge bad though because when I lived in Australia, I went to a park and there was a very friendly girl ostrich that kept following me around. I was afraid that it was going to chase and trample on me but I did not try to run away (no point in doing that because you know how fast they run). When the crowd moved on, however, I was still at the other end trying to get rid of the bird. The whole group laughed and laughed at the sight of me trying to avoid the ostrich. As it turned out, all it wanted to do was look at my gold ring. Who knew that gold, too, can make a bird go weak in the knees?

Indra

What can I say? Nicholas attracts all the 'birds', but even though this is a two-legged variety, it's still the wrong kind! Poor fella! Getting back to ostrich… from a nutritional standpoint, it truly is a healthy alternative to common meats. It's low in fat, cholesterol and calories. Yet, it's high in protein, iron, niacin, zinc and phosphorus. In short, it is a good substitute for red meats like beef or lamb in your healthy diet plan.

Nicholas has since come up with some brilliant ostrich recipes that really opened my eyes to the versatility of this new red meat.

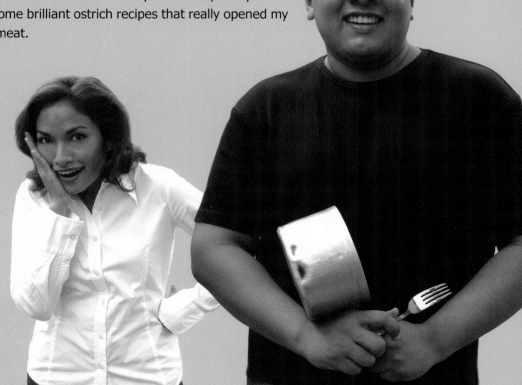

OSTRICH

PAN-GRILLED GROUND OSTRICH

Nick's culinary jottings: Although this is similar to chicken patties, the flavours differ and of course, with the use of ostrich, it is much healthier. You know this recipe is also ideal for BBQ if you like. These can be prepared overnight and left in the refrigerator. Some people freeze them but I feel the vegetables taste funny after that, so just do it the night before and leave them in the refrigerator.

Preparation time : 15 minutes
Cooking time : 20 minutes
Serves 4

Ingredients

Ostrich meat	500 g, minced
Onion	1, large, peeled and minced
Garlic	2 cloves, peeled and minced
Vietnamese mint (*daun kesum*)	30 g, roughly minced
Curry powder	1 tsp
Dried basil leaves	1 tsp
Chilli flakes	½ tsp or more to taste
Coarse black pepper	1 tsp
Dry breadcrumbs	50 g
Salt	to taste
Spray oil	

Method

- Except spray oil, combine all other ingredients in a bowl. Leave to marinate for about 1 hour.
- Shape combined ingredients into patties of desired size.
- Heat a nonstick pan. Apply some spray oil, then fry patties. Do not use high heat as the outside will burn leaving the insides raw.
- These patties can be eaten as part of a burger, in pita bread or with rice or salad.

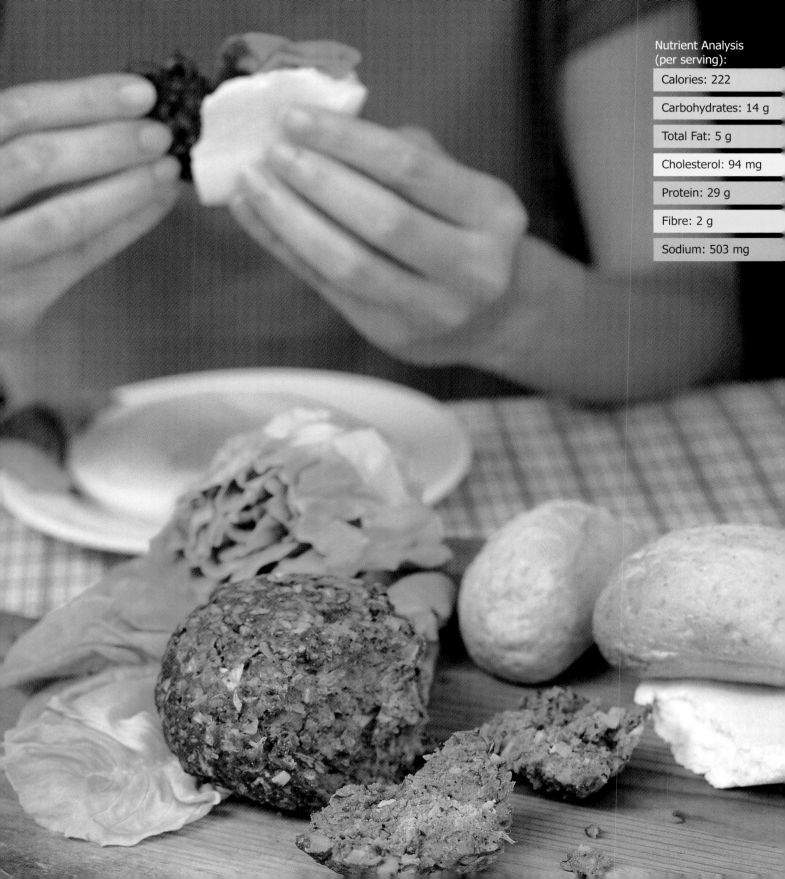

Nutrient Analysis
(per serving):

Calories: 222

Carbohydrates: 14 g

Total Fat: 5 g

Cholesterol: 94 mg

Protein: 29 g

Fibre: 2 g

Sodium: 503 mg

Nutrient Analysis
(per serving):

Calories: 227

Carbohydrates: 17 g

Total Fat: 6 g

Cholesterol: 75 mg

Protein: 25 g

Fibre: 3 g

Sodium: 224 mg

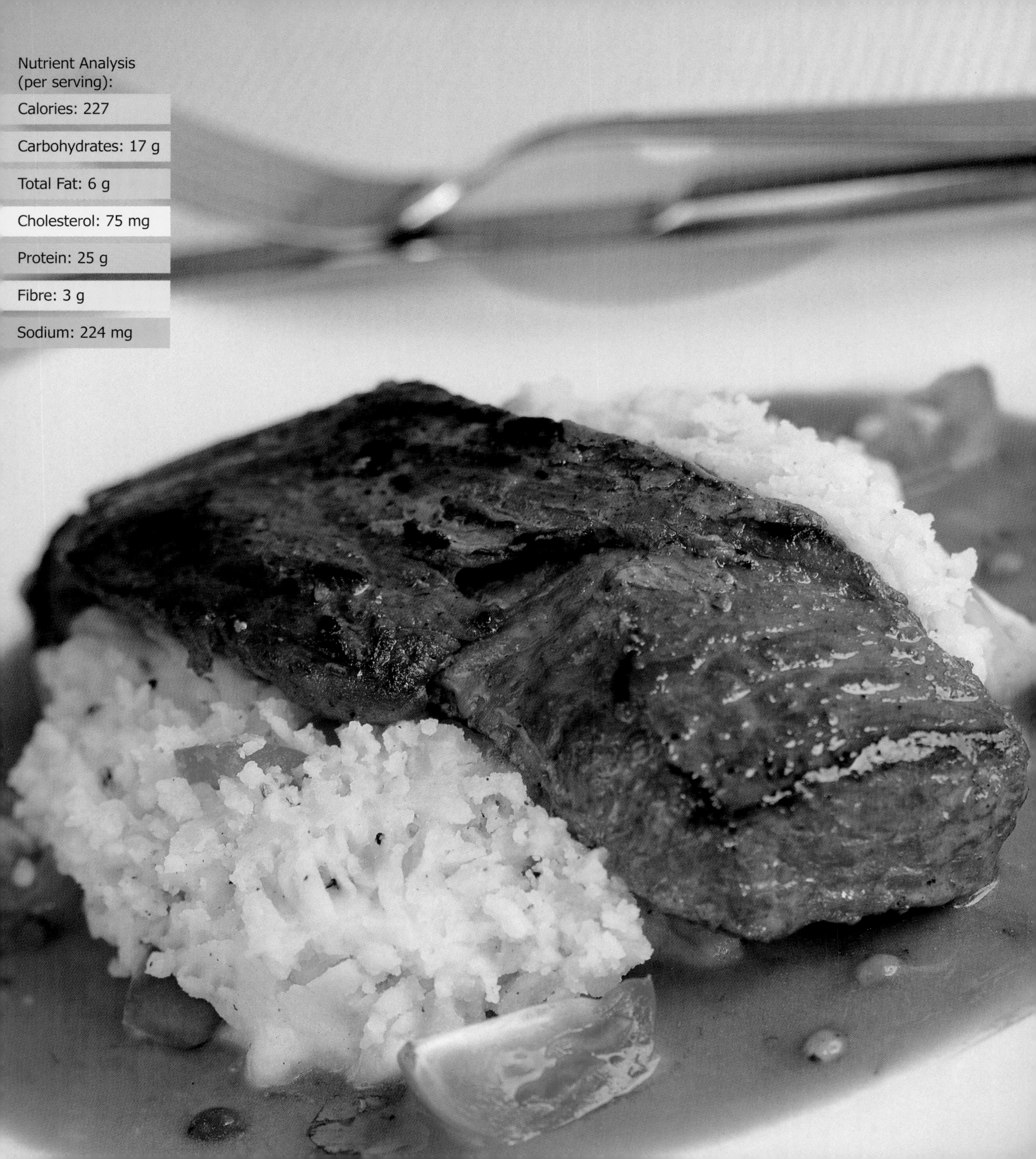

OSTRICH WITH PEPPERCORNS AND WINE SAUCE

Nick's culinary jottings: This is an easy recipe to follow and produces restaurant fare, so the next time you order something like this, hit yourself, because the recipe is here. The mixture of Asian spices together with rosemary, wine and rice milk makes this dish interestingly flavoursome.

Method

- Blend (process) peppercorns, mustard seeds, garlic and lemon grass together.

- Combine blended ingredients, sugar and meat in a large bowl. Mix well and leave aside for about 1 hour. Mix in salt only just before cooking.

- In a pot, bring rice milk to the boil. When simmering, add onion and rosemary. Leave to simmer until onions are translucent. Beat in flour.

- Lightly coat a pan with spray oil. Cook meat as you would normal steaks.

- Adjust simmering sauce to taste with salt and pepper. Increase heat, then add parsley and wine. Serve immediately with sides such as mashed potatoes or salad of your choice.

Preparation time : 15 minutes
Cooking time : 20 minutes (cook meat and sauce simultaneously)

Serves 5

Ingredients

Black peppercorns	32 g
Mustard seeds	16 g
Garlic	4 cloves
Lemon grass (*serai*)	2 stalks
Sugar	1 pinch
Ostrich steaks	5, about 100 g each
Salt	to taste
Spray oil	

Wine sauce

Rice milk	250 ml
Onion	1, small, peeled and minced
Dried rosemary	$\frac{1}{2}$ tsp
Plain (all-purpose) flour	2 Tbsp
Salt and pepper	to taste
Chopped parsley	60 g
Red wine (sweet wine of your taste)	125 ml

SPICYOSTRICHKEBABS

Nick's culinary jottings: This easy party dish can be made in a few minutes. It can be done well ahead of time, say the night before and then skewered the next day. It is a good idea to marinate the vegetables you will be using to skewer to add flavour to the kebab. Actually, you can pick any hardy vegetable of your choice to skewer with the meat.

Preparation time : 15 minutes
Cooking time : 20 minutes
Serves 4

Ingredients

Ostrich meat	500 g, to be cut into thick strips
Onions	10, small, peeled
Pineapple	1, sweet, peeled and cut into bite-size cubes
Cherry tomatoes	1 punnet
Bamboo skewers	8–10, soaked in water
Spray oil	

Marinade

Soy milk	125 ml
Black pepper	1 tsp
Sweet basil leaves	60 g, finely chopped
Paprika (less spicy)	2 tsp
Garlic	2 cloves, peeled and crushed
Salt	to taste

Method

- Combine marinade ingredients in a large bowl. Add meat, onions, pineapple and tomatoes. Mix well, then leave to marinate.
- Skewer as shown.
- Apply spray oil onto a nonstick pan. Cook kebabs until done. Each sizzling lot should take about 5 minutes to cook.

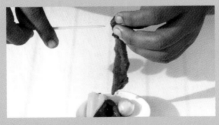 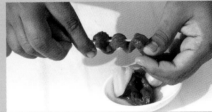

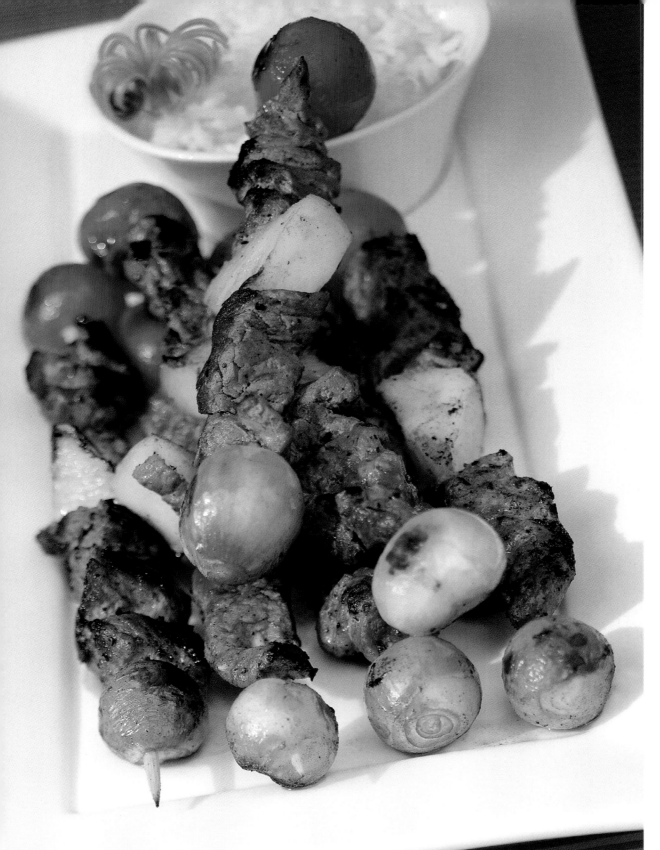

Nutrient Analysis (per serving):

Calories: 253

Carbohydrates: 22 g

Total Fat: 5 g

Cholesterol: 94 mg

Protein: 31 g

Fibre: 5 g

Sodium: 297 mg

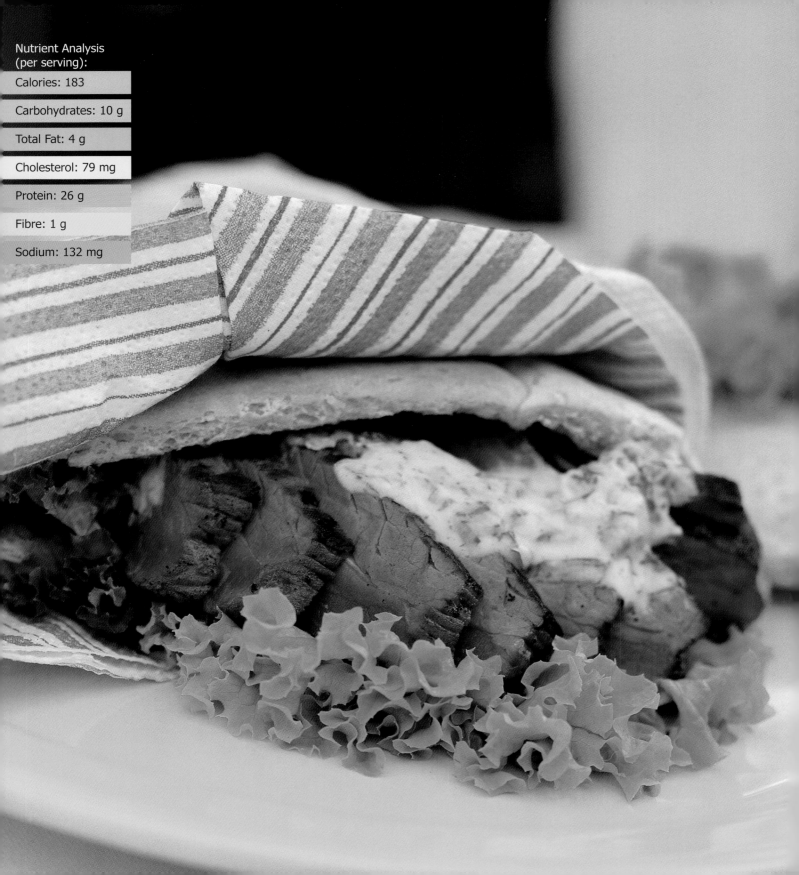

Nutrient Analysis
(per serving):

Calories: 183

Carbohydrates: 10 g

Total Fat: 4 g

Cholesterol: 79 mg

Protein: 26 g

Fibre: 1 g

Sodium: 132 mg

OSTRICHMURGH

Nick's culinary jottings: Ostrich *murgh* may not sound very nice, as Indra has attested with a funny-sounding voice, but the end result just speaks for itself. It is much healthier than using chicken and is not as dry and much tastier, I feel. Ostrich is just a wonderful meat to work with.

Method

- Except meat and spray oil, combine all other ingredients in a large bowl. Add meat and leave to marinate, preferably overnight.

- Heat a nonstick pan. Apply spray oil. Cook steaks over medium heat, turning after 3–4 minutes of sizzling.

- Steaks may be eaten with rice or with similarly flat breads like pita, *naan* and *lavash*. Also, don't forget your salads.

Preparation time : 20 minutes
Cooking time : 20 minutes
Serves 5

Ingredients

Garlic	4 cloves, peeled and minced
Minced ginger	2 Tbsp
Onion	1, peeled and coarsely chopped
Plain low-fat yoghurt	340 g
Ground cardamom	2 tsp
Chopped coriander	60 g
Chaat masala	1 Tbsp
Lemon juice	to taste
Salt and pepper	to taste
Ostrich steaks	5, about 100 g each
Spray oil	2 squirts

Nicholas

You know, the importance of pork in our community was really stressed when the nipah virus struck a few years ago. I never ever knew it was a billion-dollar industry but it is. During that time, many Chinese were all out to give pork a second chance. I witnessed pork parties, roast pork-cutting ceremonies... gosh, it was pork all the way.

While I still cannot look at pork as being the other white meat, I guess it does have some features that cannot be found in other meats. I do not consume very much pork for some reason, however a good side of bacon and ham can tickle my fancy on most occasions. My Aunty Mary, on the other hand, will swear by pork. If she feels sick, wave a piece of pork in front of her and I believe she will get all better. It is really nice to see her enjoying it, you know. In fact, she enjoys it so much that mum has days when everything has pork in it just for Aunty Mary's sake.

Indra

Hmm, this is the first time I've ever heard of someone using pork to cure distress. Then again, any culinary story from Nicholas doesn't surprise me. He literally has me in stitches every time he goes off on a tangent when a certain food prompts his mind about some story. As for me, I doubt I'll use pork to cure my headaches. I'll stick to my usual *minyak cap kapak* (Note to the uninitiated: that is a eucalyptus oil/menthol concoction that you apply to your temples. It is rather pungent, however, so you are likely to either love it or hate it!)

One thing that pork is good for is being one of nature's best sources of Vitamin D. This vitamin is also known as the 'sunshine vitamin' because your skin synthesizes it from being exposed to the sun. Vitamin D works in tandem with the mineral calcium to keep your bones in tiptop condition.

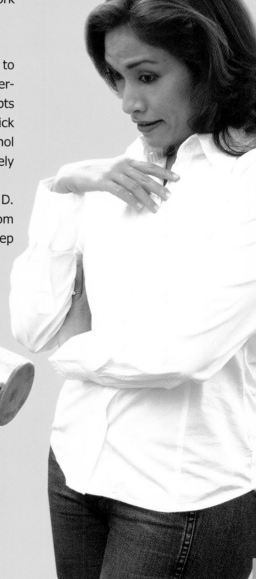

PORK

BAKEDFOOPEIKUIN

Nick's culinary jottings: This is another one of my morsel dishes, as it were. Dim sum is one of my all-time favourite meals as it comes in small morsels, just the way I like to eat my food. It is always richly laden with fat, however, and in fact, fat is sometimes purposely added so that it will remain moist. Worst of all, more oil is layered on to make it appear glossy, so for a person trying to lose weight, eating dim sum, however small the quantity, is a real no-no. One thing is for sure though, making your own dim sum will certainly cut away the variety.

Preparation time : 20 minutes
Cooking time : 20 minutes
Serves 4

Ingredients

Lean pork	300 g, minced
Salt	20 g
Corn flour (cornstarch)	20 g
Prawn (shrimp) meat	200 g
Sugar	1 tsp
Pepper	20 g
Spring onions (scallions)	20 g, finely diced
Carrots	50 g, finely diced
Sesame seed oil	20 ml
Soft bean curd skin (*foo pei*)	500 g, cut into 5-cm squares
Spray oil	

Method

- Blend (process) pork with salt until starchy. Add corn flour and blend further to combine.

- Add prawn meat, sugar and pepper. Blend to your desired texture. Transfer to a bowl.

- Add spring onions, carrots and sesame seed oil. Mix thoroughly (do not blend).

- Preheat oven to 200°C (400°F).

- To make a roll, take a piece of bean curd skin and position it such that it is a square looking on. Put a length of filling 2 cm from bottom edge. Fold in left and right edges, then roll up Swiss-roll style. Repeat until skins are used up.

- Apply 1 squirt of spray oil onto baking tray. Arrange rolls on top with seams facing downward, pressing against tray. This is so that rolls do not open up while baking. Give another spray.

- Put tray into oven. Turn rolls from time to time. Rolls should cook in about 10 minutes.

- Alternatively, you may steam the rolls, minus the oil.

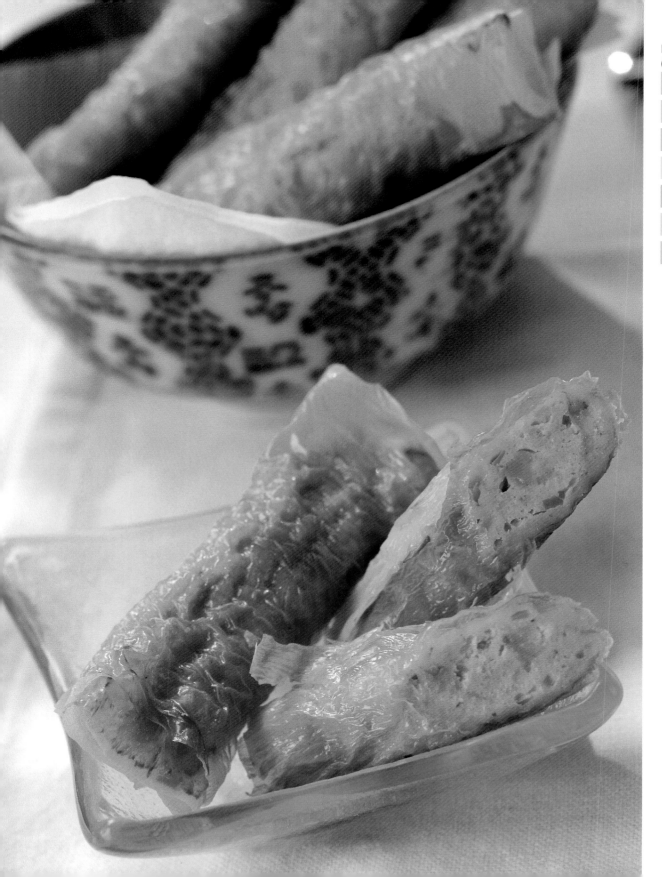

Nutrient Analysis
(per serving):

Calories: 543

Carbohydrates: 24 g

Total Fat: 25 g

Cholesterol: 106 mg

Protein: 54 g

Fibre: 2 g

Sodium: 744 mg

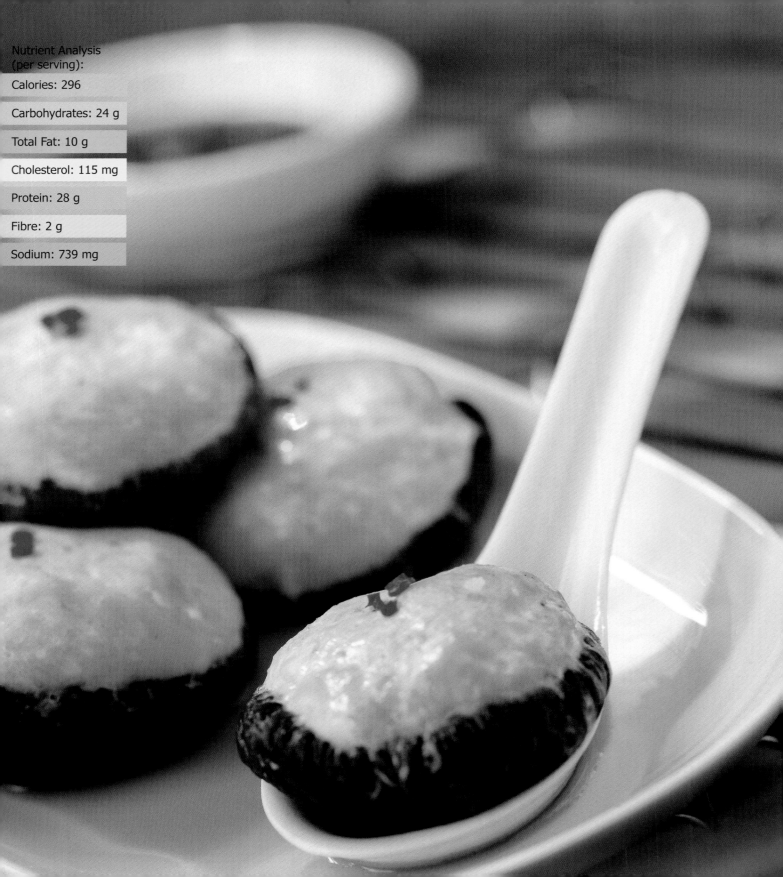

Nutrient Analysis
(per serving):

Calories: 296

Carbohydrates: 24 g

Total Fat: 10 g

Cholesterol: 115 mg

Protein: 28 g

Fibre: 2 g

Sodium: 739 mg

MUSHROOM DUMPLINGS WITH CRABMEAT

Nick's culinary jottings: This is another dim sum sort of dish. I used to enjoy watching my Chinese neighbours make them for a celebration. The women used to sit in the back of the house, with my mum usually there too, to do this and I sometimes helped them decorate the dumplings with the tiny chilli bits as I had small fingers back then, when I was also known as *ah bee bee chai.*

Preparation time : 20 minutes
Cooking time : 10 minutes
Serves 5

Method

- Except mushrooms and chilli, blend (process) all other ingredients to a moist paste.
- Stuff the underside of each mushroom until a mound forms. Repeat until mushrooms are used up.
- When done, steam for 10–15 minutes.
- Garnish with chilli bits.

Ingredients

Lean pork	300 g, minced
Corn flour (cornstarch)	10 g
Fresh prawns (shrimps)	200 g, peeled and deveined
Crabmeat	100 g
Sugar	1 tsp
Sesame seed oil	30 ml
Pepper	20 g
Spring onions (scallions)	50 g, thinly sliced
Salt	to taste
Dried Chinese mushrooms	30 g, soaked to soften, stems discarded and left whole
Red chilli	1, cut into tiny squares for garnishing

OLD-FASHIONED PORK CHOPS

Nick's culinary jottings: This is a favourite that goes back way, way before yesteryears. Usually found in Eurasian households, this was the once-in-a-while, European-influenced dish, albeit the only thing European about it was the potatoes and vegetables. While the old version was always deep-fried, this version is pan-fried. The sauce is the very essence of this dish. Back in the good, old days, when fat was not something you worried about, lard was used to sauté all the ingredients before thickening.

Preparation time : 20 minutes (not including marinating time)
Cooking time : 20–30 minutes
Serves 4

Ingredients

HP sauce	3 Tbsp
Garlic	3–4 cloves, peeled and minced
Mustard	1 Tbsp
Red wine	125 ml
Salt and pepper	to taste
Fat-free pork steaks	500 g, cut into 0.75-cm thickness and flattened with back of cleaver
Spray oil	2 squirts
Breadcrumbs	

Sauce

Onion	1, large, peeled and sliced
Tomatoes	2, large, coarsely chopped
Plain (all-purpose) flour	1 Tbsp
Stock	250 ml
Soy milk	250 ml
Black pepper	1 tsp
Salt	to taste

Method

- To make marinade, combine HP sauce, garlic, mustard and red wine. Add salt and pepper to taste, then meat. Marinate pork for a few hours.
- Heat a nonstick pan. Apply spray oil.
- Coat pork chops with breadcrumbs. Pan-fry a few at a time, turning from time to time. When done, remove and set aside. Reserve leftover marinade.
- In a dry pot, sauté onion until slightly brown. Add tomatoes and leftover marinade. Add flour and stir through. Add stock. Leave to simmer.
- Add soy milk and seasonings. Simmer for a few minutes more. Serve with your favourite vegetables or a nice, wholesome salad.

Nicholas' Tip: If alcohol is not your thing, then replace red wine with 125 ml apple juice.

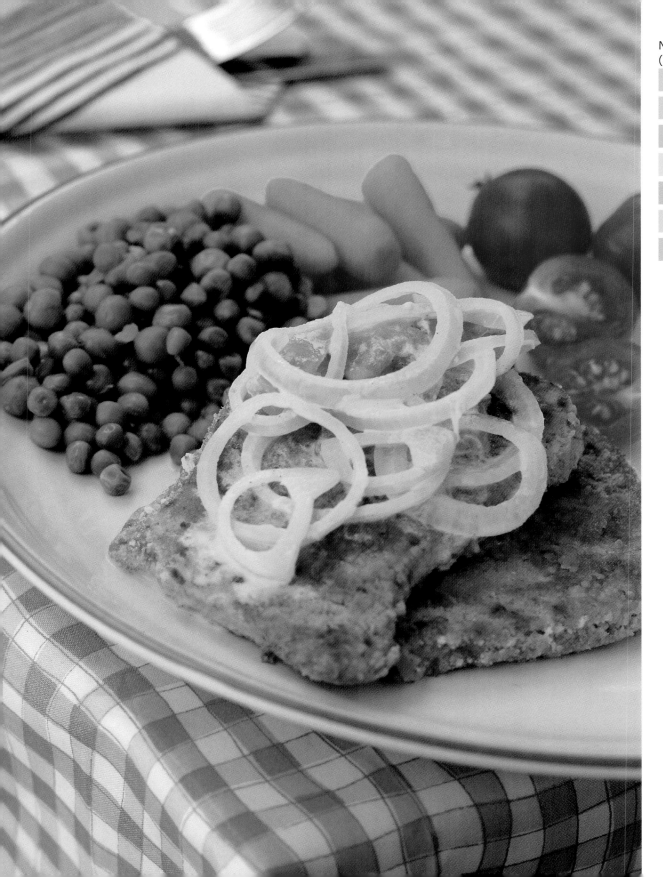

Nutrient Analysis
(per serving):

Calories: 362

Carbohydrates: 33 g

Total Fat: 9 g

Cholesterol: 76 mg

Protein: 34 g

Fibre: 4 g

Sodium: 510 mg

Nutrient Analysis
(per serving):

Calories: 220

Carbohydrates: 11 g

Total Fat: 7 g

Cholesterol: 76 mg

Protein: 28 g

Fibre: 1 g

Sodium: 236 mg

Nutrient Analysis
(per serving of sauce):

Calories: 401

Carbohydrates: 32 g

Total Fat: 27 g

Cholesterol: 0 mg

Protein: 14 g

Fibre: 5 g

Sodium: 157 mg

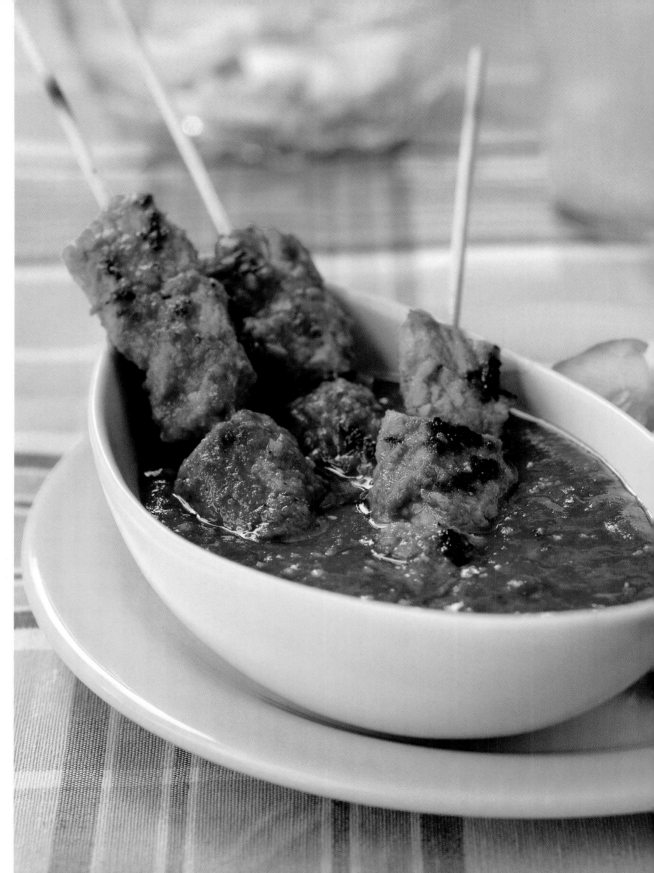

PORKSATAY

Nick's culinary jottings: As a young child, I would often wonder how pork would taste as *satay*. Funnily enough, I never ventured to try it until it was bought one day and no one told me what it was. It was succulent and I have to say a lot better tasting than chicken and beef. One tip here is not to expect the *satay* to be glistening and succulent looking when it's done because the traditional way of grilling it is to smother it with heaps of oil and sugar.

Preparation time : 20–30 minutes
Cooking time   : 30 minutes
Serves 4

Method

- Blend (process) onions, garlic, galangal, lemon grass and ginger together.

- To make marinade, combine blended ingredients, ground coriander, cumin, sugar and salt to taste. Marinate pork for about 20–30 minutes.

- Skewer a few pieces of meat onto one stick. Repeat until meat is used up. Leave for 1 hour or longer if desired.

- Preheat oven to 180°C (200°F).

- Line a tray with tin foil. Arrange *satay* on top. Cover with foil and bake for a while. Turn once or twice.

- Set oven to grill. Remove tin foil cover. Grill for a few minutes until done. Serve with peanut sauce if desired.

- To make peanut sauce, first blend (process) onion, garlic, galangal, lemon grass and red chillies together.

- Combine blended ingredients, palm sugar and tamarind juice in a pot. Simmer for about 30 minutes for flavours to infuse.

- Add peanuts, salt and soy milk if used. Let it thicken.

Ingredients

Onions	2, large, peeled
Garlic	3 cloves, peeled
Galangal (*lengkuas*)	100 g, peeled
Lemon grass (*serai*)	6 stalks
Ginger	50 g, peeled
Ground coriander (cilantro)	2 Tbsp
Cumin	1 Tbsp
Sugar	3 Tbsp
Salt	to taste
Lean pork	500 g, cut into 2-cm chunks
Skewers	

Peanut sauce

Onion	1, peeled
Garlic	2–3 cloves, peeled
Galangal (*lengkuas*)	50 g, peeled
Lemon grass (*serai*)	3 stalks
Red chillies	2–3
Palm sugar (*gula Melaka*)	200 g, melted in boiling water and strained for grit
Tamarind (*asam Jawa*) juice	250 ml
Peanuts (groundnuts)	220 g, toasted and coarsely ground
Salt	to taste
Soy milk (optional)	to taste

CAMBODIANPORKWITHLIMESAUCE

Nick's culinary jottings: When I ate this the first time, I really did not enjoy it because it was really fatty pork that the seller used. The taste was nice but the meat was a real waste. This simple pan-fried pork dish is easy to make and the meat can be marinated and kept in the freezer for ages. I have added some capsicum, carrots and mushrooms to make this a one-pot wonder.

Preparation time : 20 minutes
Cooking time : 30 minutes
Serves 5

Ingredients

Garlic	6–7 cloves, peeled and minced
Black pepper	1 Tbsp
Sugar	2 tsp
Lemon juice	3 Tbsp
Ginger	30 g, peeled and sliced
Fish sauce	to taste
Fat-free pork steaks	500 g, cut into stir-fry strips
Onion	1, peeled and minced
Stock	250 ml
Dried Chinese mushrooms	10, soaked to soften, stems discarded and boiled until partially cooked
Carrot	1, peeled if desired and sliced any way you like
Ground white pepper	to taste
Green capsicum (sweet bell pepper)	2, cut into bite-size pieces
Corn flour (cornstarch)	1/2 Tbsp, mixed with a little water to make thickener

Method

- To make marinade, combine garlic, black pepper, sugar, lemon juice, ginger and fish sauce to taste. Marinate pork for a few minutes.

- In dry pan, sauté onion until light brown. Add stock, then mushrooms and simmer.

- Add marinated pork and carrot. Cook over low heat for about 10–15 minutes.

- Season to taste with white pepper and more fish sauce if desired. Bring to the boil. Add capsicum. Leave to boil for 2 minutes.

- Add corn flour mixture to thicken. Serve with rice.

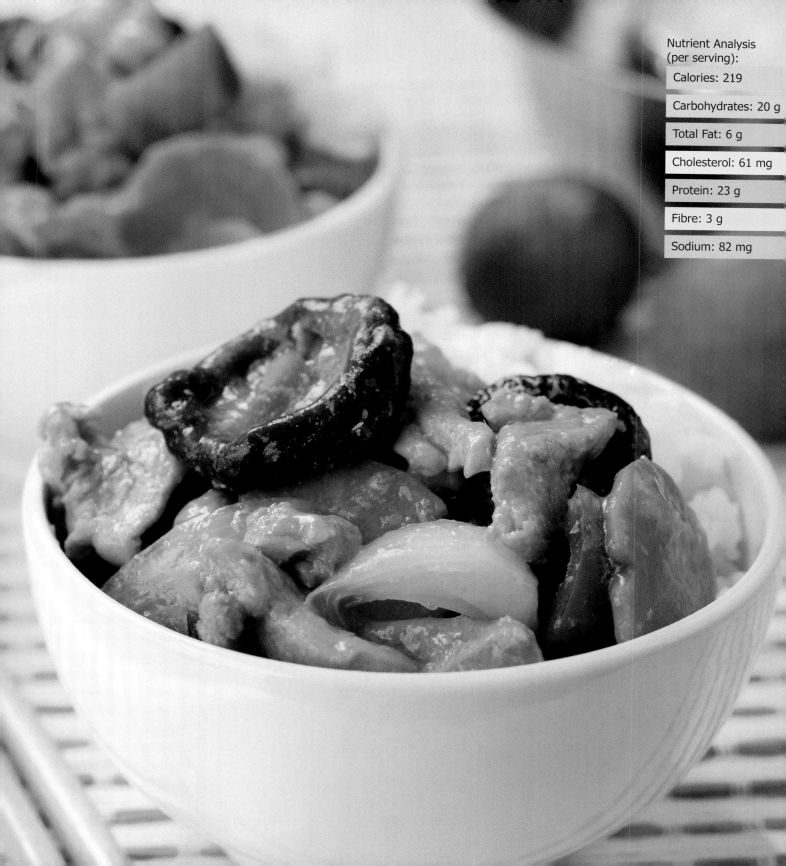

Nutrient Analysis
(per serving):

Calories: 219

Carbohydrates: 20 g

Total Fat: 6 g

Cholesterol: 61 mg

Protein: 23 g

Fibre: 3 g

Sodium: 82 mg

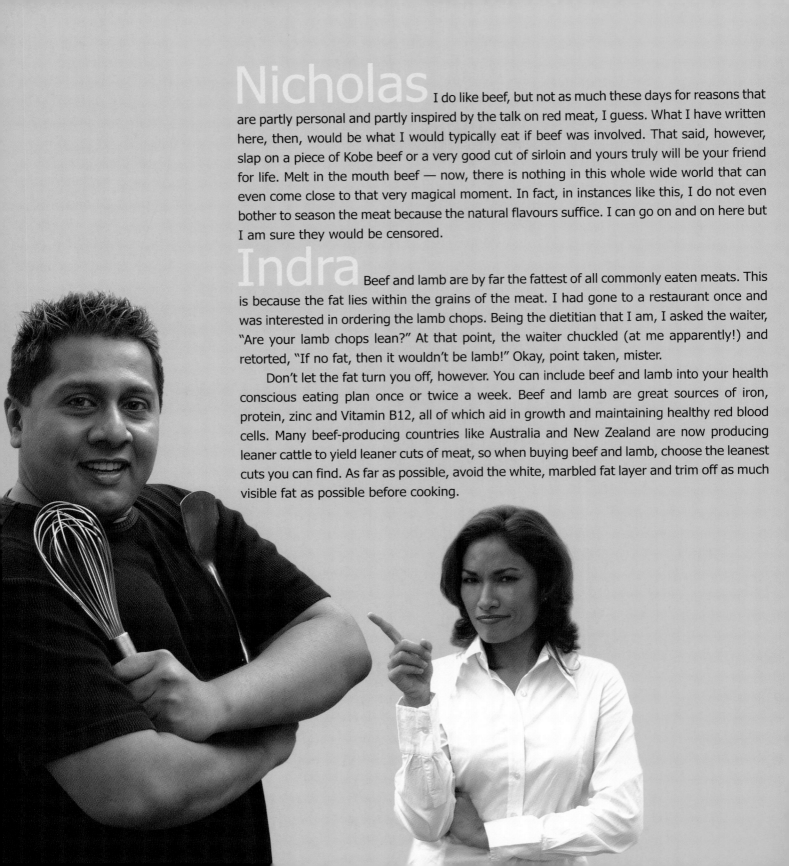

Nicholas

I do like beef, but not as much these days for reasons that are partly personal and partly inspired by the talk on red meat, I guess. What I have written here, then, would be what I would typically eat if beef was involved. That said, however, slap on a piece of Kobe beef or a very good cut of sirloin and yours truly will be your friend for life. Melt in the mouth beef — now, there is nothing in this whole wide world that can even come close to that very magical moment. In fact, in instances like this, I do not even bother to season the meat because the natural flavours suffice. I can go on and on here but I am sure they would be censored.

Indra

Beef and lamb are by far the fattest of all commonly eaten meats. This is because the fat lies within the grains of the meat. I had gone to a restaurant once and was interested in ordering the lamb chops. Being the dietitian that I am, I asked the waiter, "Are your lamb chops lean?" At that point, the waiter chuckled (at me apparently!) and retorted, "If no fat, then it wouldn't be lamb!" Okay, point taken, mister.

Don't let the fat turn you off, however. You can include beef and lamb into your health conscious eating plan once or twice a week. Beef and lamb are great sources of iron, protein, zinc and Vitamin B12, all of which aid in growth and maintaining healthy red blood cells. Many beef-producing countries like Australia and New Zealand are now producing leaner cattle to yield leaner cuts of meat, so when buying beef and lamb, choose the leanest cuts you can find. As far as possible, avoid the white, marbled fat layer and trim off as much visible fat as possible before cooking.

BEEF AND LAMB

BEEFSTEW

Nick's culinary jottings: Beef stew is a favourite in most communities in this world. It is rich and keeps you warm, and leaves a wonderful aroma wafting in your kitchen. Remember that stews and some soups are always better the next day.

Preparation time : 30 minutes
Cooking time : 60 minutes
Serves 5

Ingredients

Spray oil	2–3 squirts
Stewing beef	1 kg, excess fat trimmed off
Plain (all purpose) flour	60 g
Stock	750 ml
Garlic	2 cloves
Tomatoes	3, large, coarsely chopped
Bay leaves	2
Oregano	1 tsp
Onions	2, large, peeled and cut into wedges
Baby potatoes	10, washed, brushed clean, and with skins left intact
Celery	120 g, cut into bite-size pieces
Black pepper	1 tsp
Salt	to taste
Broccoli florets	370 g
French beans	200 g, cut into 3-cm long pieces

Method

- Heat a pot. Apply spray oil. Sear meat until light brown. There should be some liquid by now. Add flour and stir constantly to prevent lumps.

- Add stock, then garlic and tomatoes. Stir in bay leaves and oregano. Simmer for about 30 minutes.

- Add onions, potatoes and celery. Simmer for another 30 minutes.

- Adjust to taste with salt and pepper. When meat is tender, add broccoli and beans. Simmer for 5 minutes more.

- Serve with rice, mashed potatoes, crusty French bread or trusty toast.

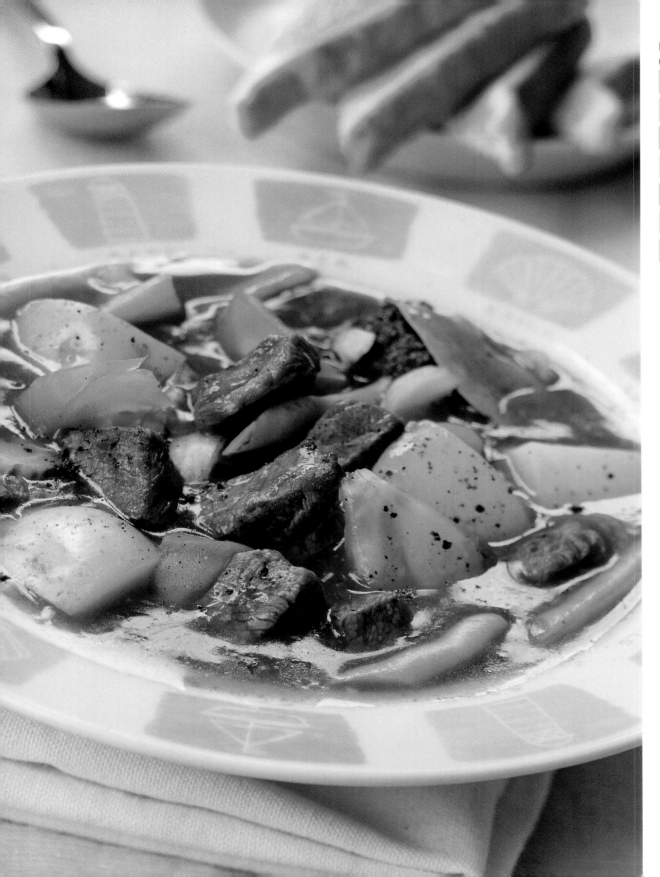

Nutrient Analysis
(per serving):

Calories: 428

Carbohydrates: 37 g

Total Fat: 9 g

Cholesterol: 74 mg

Protein: 49 g

Fibre: 33 g

Sodium: 268 mg

Nutrient Analysis
(per serving):

Calories: 270

Carbohydrates: 10 g

Total Fat: 9 g

Cholesterol: 62 mg

Protein: 37 g

Fibre: 3 g

Sodium: 206 mg

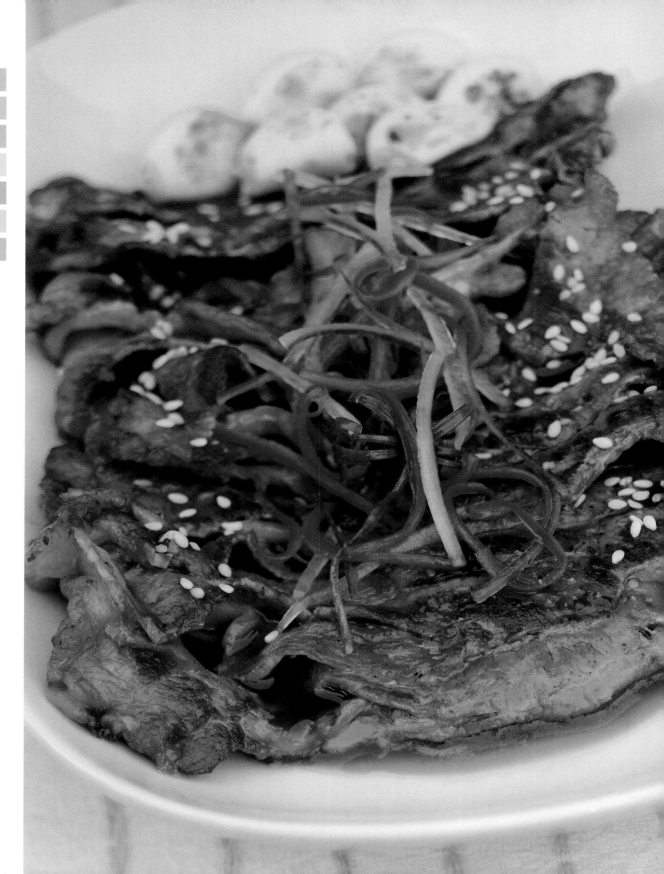

KOREAN BULGOGI

Nick's culinary jottings: My friend Kwon Mi Kyung taught me this splendid recipe. She actually could not cook when she got married but to stay in keeping with Korean cultural traditions, she learnt it real quick. There was never a day when I lived in Australia that I would not 'accidentally' plant myself at her house during dinnertime.

Preparation time : 20 minutes
Cooking time : 20–25 minutes
Serves 6

Method

- Except meat, combine all other ingredients in a bowl. Mix well. Add meat and leave to marinate overnight.

- On cooking day, preheat oven to 180°C (350°F).

- Line a tray with tin foil. Arrange meat strips neatly, and slightly overlapping to prevent drying. Cover with more foil.

- Bake for about 15 minutes. Turn meat over and bake for 3–5 minutes. Switch to grill and leave in oven for 3–4 minutes more.

- Garnish with toasted sesame seeds, as well as julienned red chilli and spring onion if used.

- For a more flavourful dish, serve with a side of roasted garlic if desired. To roast garlic, just cook them on a dry nonstick pan until golden brown.

☙ Note: If you have a nonstick cake pan, then grill the beef in the oven at 200°C (400°F) covered in foil.

Ingredients

Onion juice	extracted from 2 onions
Carrots	2, grated
Nashi pears	2, grated
Sugar	2 tsp
Sesame seed oil	2 tsp
Black pepper	1 tsp or more to taste
Salt	to taste
Scotch fillet or strip loin	1 kg, thinly sliced (never mind size, as long as it's thin)

Garnishing

Toasted sesame seeds
Julienned red chilli (optional)
Julienned spring onion (scallion) (optional)

PEPPERBEEF

Nick's culinary jottings: This is a good ol'e Eurasian favourite. In the old days, when meat was rather scarce at mealtimes, according to my mother that is, this dish was made only during birthdays and festivities. Every Eurasian household, though, would have its own recipe that would seldom or never be divulged.

Preparation time : 30 minutes
Cooking time : 45–60 minutes
Serves 5

Ingredients

Beef steaks	500 g, cut into thin slices and marinated with salt, pepper and 2 star anise
Water	500 ml
Garlic	3 cloves, peeled and roughly chopped
Onions	2, large, peeled and thickly sliced
Carrot	1, large, peeled if desired and sliced
Potatoes	2, large, peeled if desired and cut like big chips (fries), then parboiled until half-cooked; replace able with a handful of baby potatoes
Ground black pepper	2 tsp
Ground white pepper	1 tsp
Sugar	1 tsp
Salt	to taste
Green peas	160 g
Corn flour (cornstarch)	1 Tbsp, mixed with a little water to make thickener

Method

- Boil beef in water until just tender. Do not over boil.
- Add garlic, onions and carrot. Boil until liquid is reduced. Add potatoes and boil a few minutes more.
- Add peppers, sugar and salt to taste. Boil until further reduced. Add peas.
- Add corn flour mixture to thicken.
- Serve hot with rice.

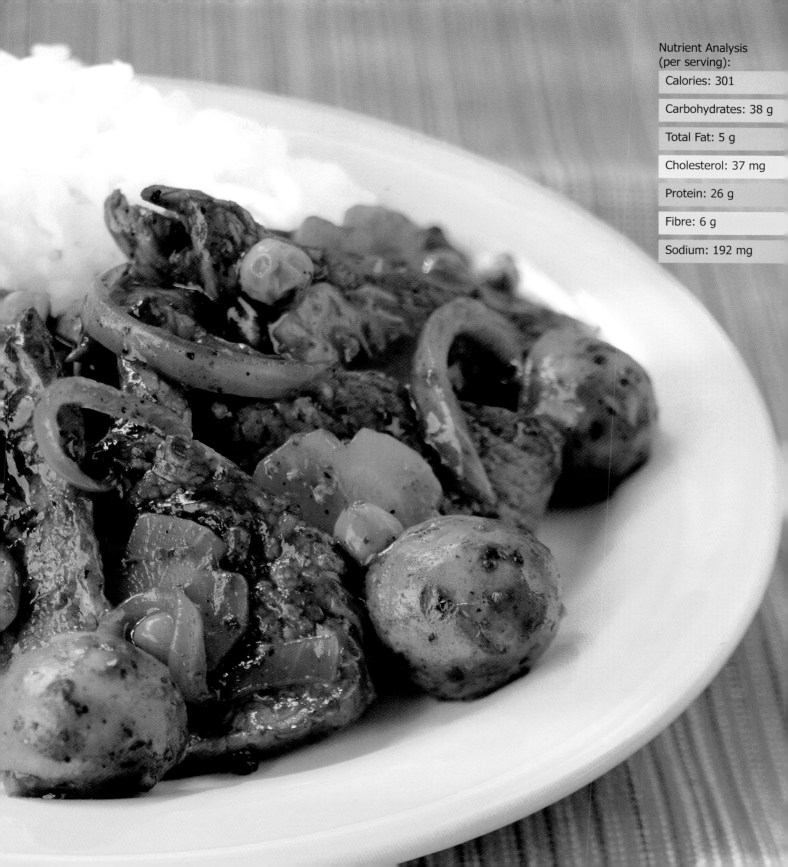

Nutrient Analysis
(per serving):

Calories: 301

Carbohydrates: 38 g

Total Fat: 5 g

Cholesterol: 37 mg

Protein: 26 g

Fibre: 6 g

Sodium: 192 mg

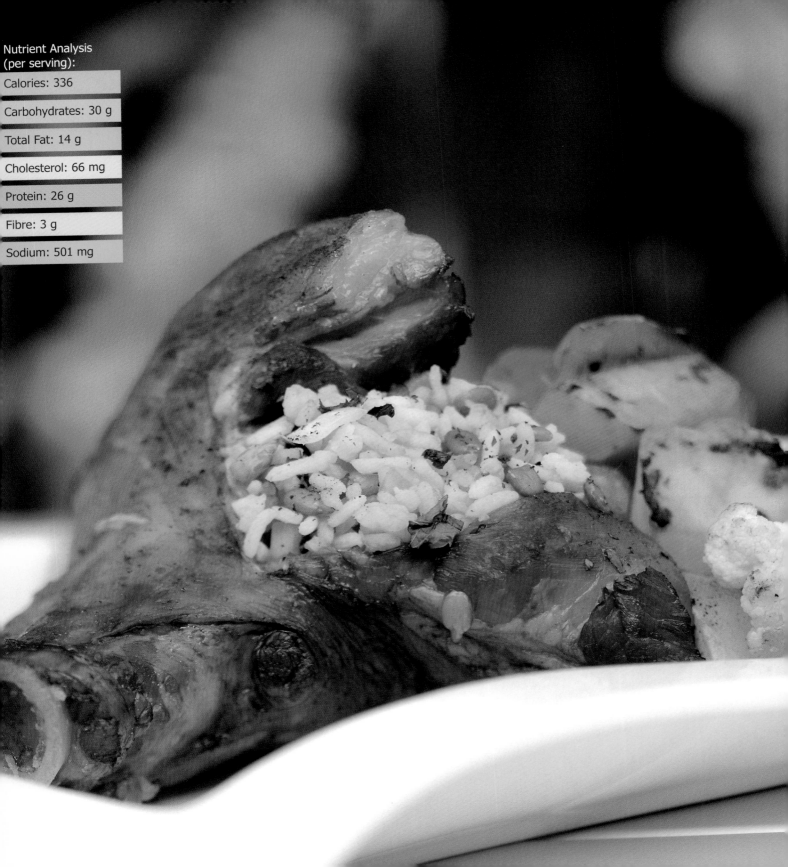

Nutrient Analysis
(per serving):

Calories: 336

Carbohydrates: 30 g

Total Fat: 14 g

Cholesterol: 66 mg

Protein: 26 g

Fibre: 3 g

Sodium: 501 mg

STUFFED LAMB SHANKS

Nick's culinary jottings: This is so easy and can be done in advance. Use leftover rice. In fact, you can stuff just about any kind of leftover food inside the lamb shanks, you know. Just don't be too smart and put in leafy vegetables from yesterday because it will wind up looking like a witch's brew.

Preparation time : 20 minutes
Cooking time : 45–60 minutes
Serves 5

Method

- Combine all marinade ingredients in a bowl. Add lamb and leave to marinate, preferably overnight.
- On cooking day, preheat oven to 180°C (350°F).
- To facilitate stuffing later, slit lamb as shown.
- Combine all remaining ingredients in a bowl to make stuffing. Mix well.
- Stuff lamb as shown, then secure with toothpicks (cocktail sticks). Place in a heatproof baking (flameproof casserole) dish and bake until done.
- Serve with vegetables of your choice.

Ingredients

Lamb shanks	5, excess fat trimmed off
Cooked rice	200 g
Onion	1, peeled and minced
Minced garlic	1 tsp
Fresh button mushrooms	160 g
Pine nuts	120 g
Parsley	30 g, minced
Salt and pepper	to taste

Marinade

Worcestershire sauce	125 ml
Black pepper	1 Tbsp
Curry powder	1 Tbsp
Minced lemon grass (*serai*)	1 Tbsp
Ketchup	5 Tbsp
Sugar	1 tsp
Onion	1, peeled and minced
Garlic	4 cloves, peeled and minced
Salt	to taste

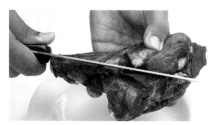
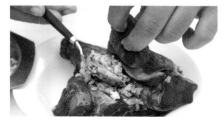
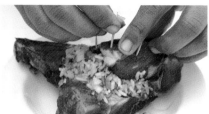

JAPANESE BEEF YAKITORI

Nick's culinary jottings: While most Japanese would just use a bottled sauce, I quite by accident came up with this, thanks to Carol Shun, my good friend and resident gourmand, because when she does not grumble about something, then we know we've got a hit! One thing to note — do not marinate for too long or the wine and *mirin* will overpower the beef after a while.

Preparation time : 15 minutes
Cooking time : 20–30 minutes
Serves 4

Ingredients

Beef fillet	500 g, cut into slightly big pieces
Bamboo skewers	10–15, soaked in water
Spring onions (scallions)	200 g, cut into 3-cm lengths
Spray oil	2 squirts
Julienned red chilli	

Marinade

Sake	125 ml
Dark soy sauce	3 Tbsp
Minced ginger	2 Tbsp
Mirin	125 ml
Sugar	2 Tbsp
Salt and pepper	to taste

Method

- Combine all marinade ingredients in a bowl. Mix well.
- Marinate beef pieces for a few minutes. Skewer them, alternating with spring onions.
- Heat a flat nonstick pan. Spray on oil. Cook skewers of meat, turning from time to time. It should take around 5 minutes per stick.
- To serve, garnish with julienned red chilli if desired.

Note: A wine made from fermented rice, *sake* is the national beverage of Japan. *Mirin*, on the other hand, is a cooking wine made from glutinous rice and has a rich golden colour.

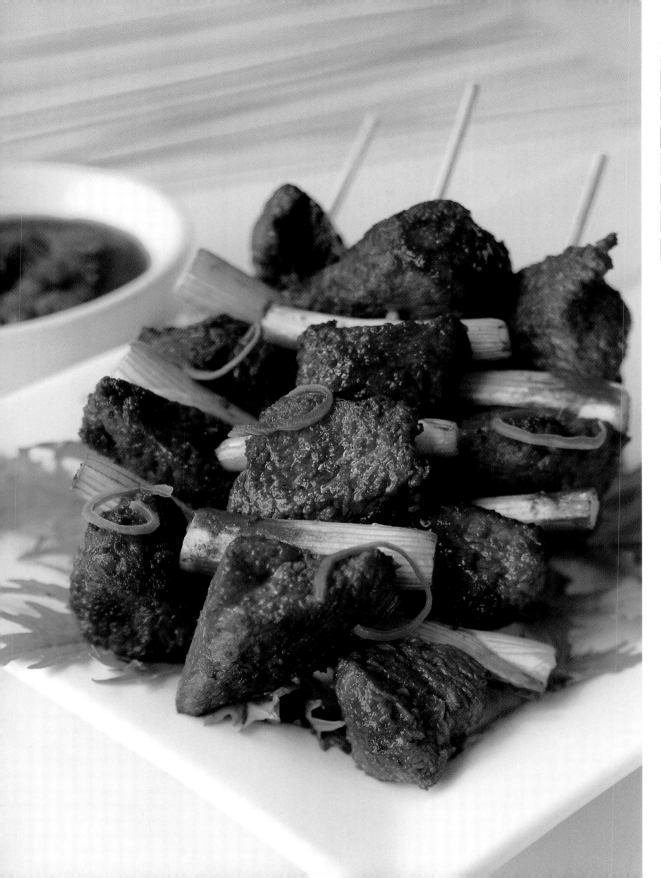

Nutrient Analysis
(per serving):

Calories: 228

Carbohydrates: 15 g

Total Fat: 5 g

Cholesterol: 46 mg

Protein: 28 g

Fibre: 2 g

Sodium: 386 mg

Nutrient Analysis
(per serving):

Calories: 165

Carbohydrates: 9 g

Total Fat: 4 g

Cholesterol: 37 mg

Protein: 22 g

Fibre: 0 g

Sodium: 172 mg

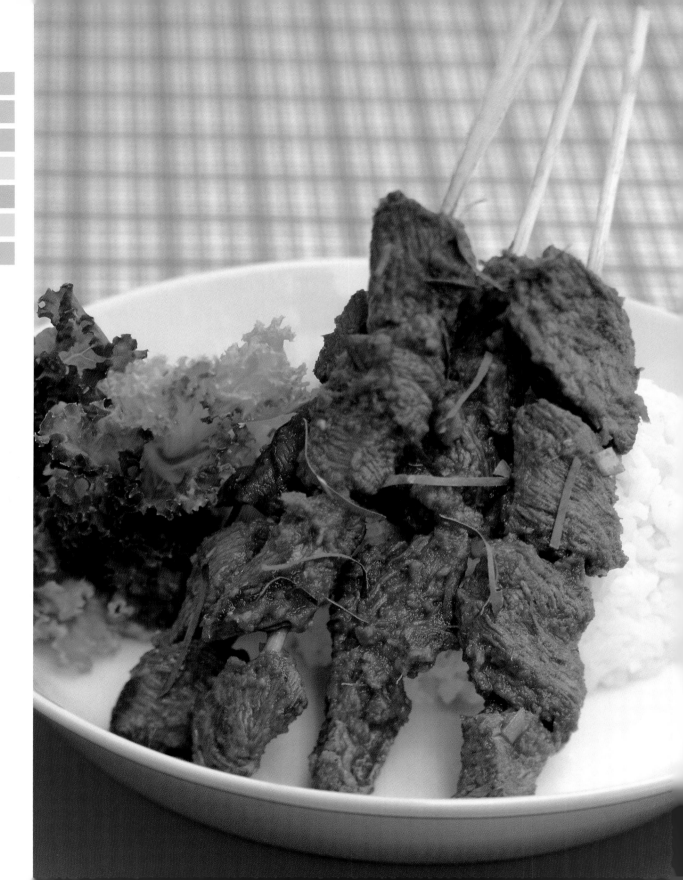

CAMBOGEE BEEF

Nick's culinary jottings: Cambogee is another version of *satay* from Cambodia. *Satay* is a dish of the Malay people that involves grilling small pieces meat on skewers over charcoal embers. For *cambogee*, the marinade is boiled before it is poured over the meat and the result is oh-so-tender pieces of meat. Marinate meat overnight before skewering it so that it is at its most flavourful.

Preparation time : 20–30 minutes
Cooking time : 60 minutes
Serves 5

Method

- Except meat, boil all other ingredients in a pot. Taste to test if done; it should be slightly sweet but not overpowering.
- Pour boiled ingredients over meat. Leave to marinate overnight.
- On cooking day, soak some bamboo skewers in water. Skewer meat pieces, then grill over low heat. High heat will cause sugar to burn.
- Serve with rice and salad of your choice.
- Use leftover marinade as a sauce if desired. Simmer until liquid is halved. Add more chillies for a spicier sauce.

Ingredients

Kaffir lime leaves	8, very thinly sliced
Lemon grass (*serai*)	6 stalks, blended (processed)
Galangal (*lengkuas*)	50 g, peeled and blended (processed)
Red chillies	2–3, blended (processed)
Garlic	5 cloves, peeled and blended (processed)
Sugar	2–3 Tbsp
Stock	500 ml
Light soy sauce	to taste
Beef steaks	500 g, cut into large bite-size pieces

AAB-GOOSHT-E BAADENJAAN

Nick's culinary jottings: I tasted this Iranian dish in a restaurant overseas. Funnily enough, it was in a Turkish restaurant, so I thought it was a Turkish dish until I talked about it to a friend from Turkey and he promptly replied that I was getting my foods mixed up. I sometimes wonder why restaurants try to fool us.

Preparation time : 30 minutes
Cooking time : 45 minutes
Serves 6

Ingredients

Boneless lean lamb	500 g, cut into bite-size chunks and with fat trimmed off
Channa dhal	160 g, soaked
Garlic	4 cloves, peeled and minced
Stock	750 ml
Onions	4, large, peeled and thinly sliced
Potatoes	5, peeled if desired and quartered
Tomatoes	3, large, coarsely chopped
Black pepper	to taste
Salt	to taste
Aubergines (eggplants)	3, large, cut to 0.5-cm thick slices

Method

- Sear meat in a pot until it appears cooked. Add dhal, garlic and stock. Cover with a snug-fitting lid. Simmer for about 30 minutes.

- Add onions, and potatoes and tomatoes. Adjust to taste with pepper and salt.

- Add aubergines and simmer for about 20 minutes or until cooked.

- This stew is seldom eaten with rice. Serve it with different breads.

Note: *Channa* dhal consists of skinned and split yellow peas that are a relative of the chickpea.

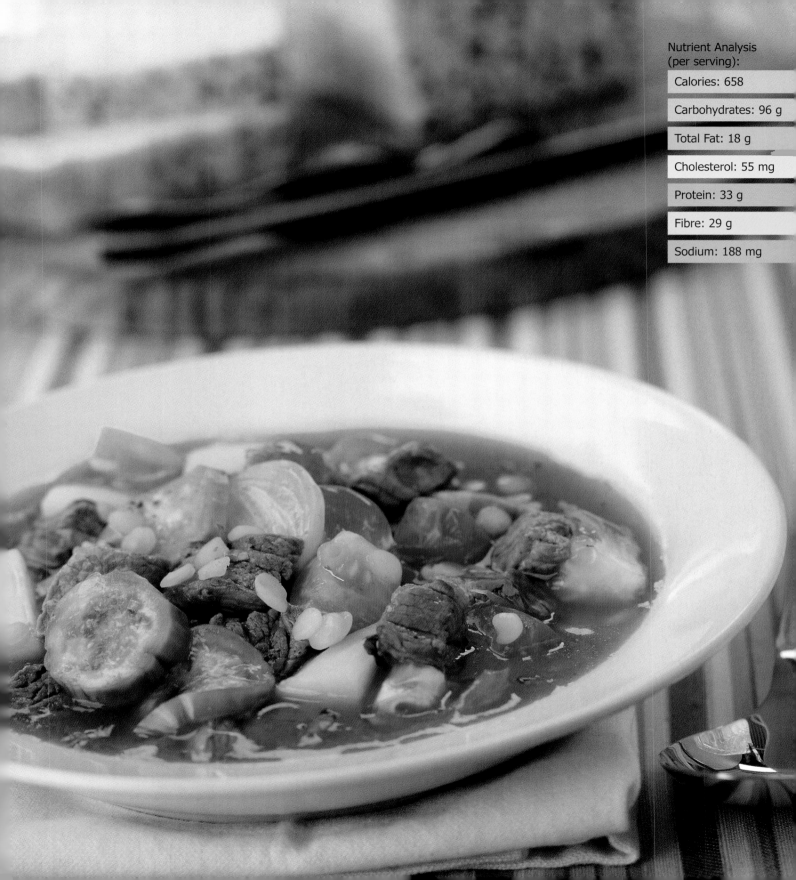

Nutrient Analysis
(per serving):

Calories: 658

Carbohydrates: 96 g

Total Fat: 18 g

Cholesterol: 55 mg

Protein: 33 g

Fibre: 29 g

Sodium: 188 mg

Nicholas

I am not really a fan of seafood, so what you see here is pretty much what I would eat if someone served them up to me. I don't know what it is with seafood but it always conjures up greed in many. During some of my catering assignments or even parties, I see people rushing if seafood is served. This does not only happen in Malaysia okay, the greedy seafood phenomenon is everywhere.

It's awful to be writing a cookbook and then telling you that I do not like certain kinds of foods, but I will only eat seafood if it is not messy; if the fish is filleted, the prawns peeled and all that jazz. That's why I always try to have mum there when I eat seafood. I am a lazy eater, I do not like to get my fingers dirty when I eat. With crab, for example, I only eat parts that can be dug out with my fork, the rest goes to mum. Also, it's a good practice when you boys go on dates. I reckon women just love it when they get to peel the prawns and shell the crab for you. I think it gives them a sense of motherliness when they do it for us... okay, I can feel that Indra's face has changed, so let's see what she says.

Indra

Nicholas, you really don't know what you're missing out on by not liking seafood. They are rich in an abundance of nutrients, including protein, selenium, iodine, zinc, Vitamin B12 and iron to name a few. Deep-sea fish such as mackerel, tuna, salmon, sea bass etc. also have Omega-3 fatty acids, which are a type of polyunsaturated fat, and research has shown that Omega-3 helps to combat coronary heart disease, arthritis and other ailments.

Seafood has a bad reputation because many people eat it in restaurants where the portions are large, and the dishes are oily and heavy (think English fish and chips or Chinese chilli crabs). Now that you know the wonderful nutritional oomph of seafood, however, maybe you'll be sure to include it more often in your meals at home. Sorry Nicholas, but I'm not going to peel those prawns for you, dear!

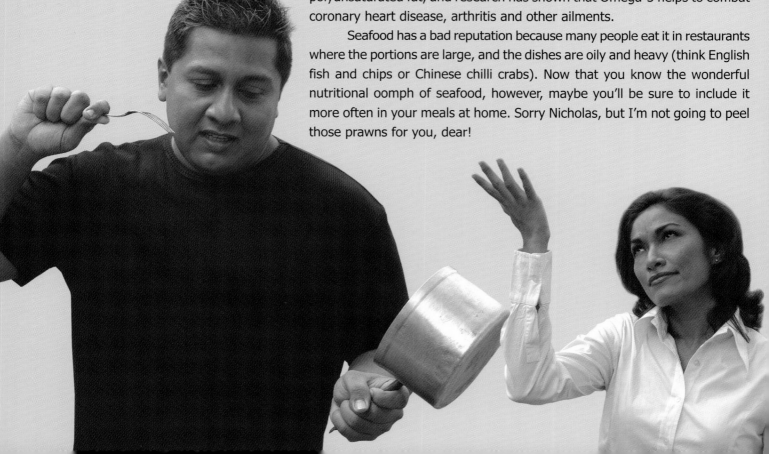

SEAFOOD

IKANBAKAR

Nick's culinary jottings: Ikan bakar is an all-time favourite with many Malaysians. During the month of Ramadan, the stall with the wafting smoke and the aroma of fish would be one with the longest line. You can put it on the barbecue or bake it in the oven. One thing is for sure, your guests won't forget it. I am fussy, too, when it comes to handling fish and sliced fish or better still, boneless fish suits me fine.

Preparation time : 20 minutes
Cooking time : 25–30 minutes
Serves 5

Ingredients

Mackerel fillets	5, about 160 g each
Banana leaves for wrapping	

Marinade

Red chillies	3
Candlenuts (*buah keras*)	5
Onions	3, large, peeled
Galangal (*lengkuas*)	50 g, peeled
Lemon grass (*serai*)	5 stalks
Thick tamarind (*asam Jawa*) juice	125 ml
Sugar	1 tsp or more to taste
Salt	to taste

Method

- Blend (process) marinade ingredients until fine. Transfer to a large bowl. Add fish and mix. Leave to marinate, preferably overnight.
- On cooking day, wrap fish with banana leaves and tin foil as shown.
- Preheat oven to 200°C (400°F).
- Bake fish for 20–25 minutes.
- Switch oven to grill and leave for 5–10 minutes more. Do not burn.

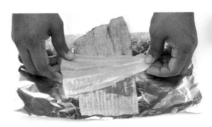
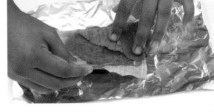
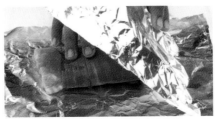
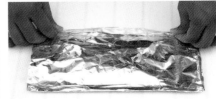

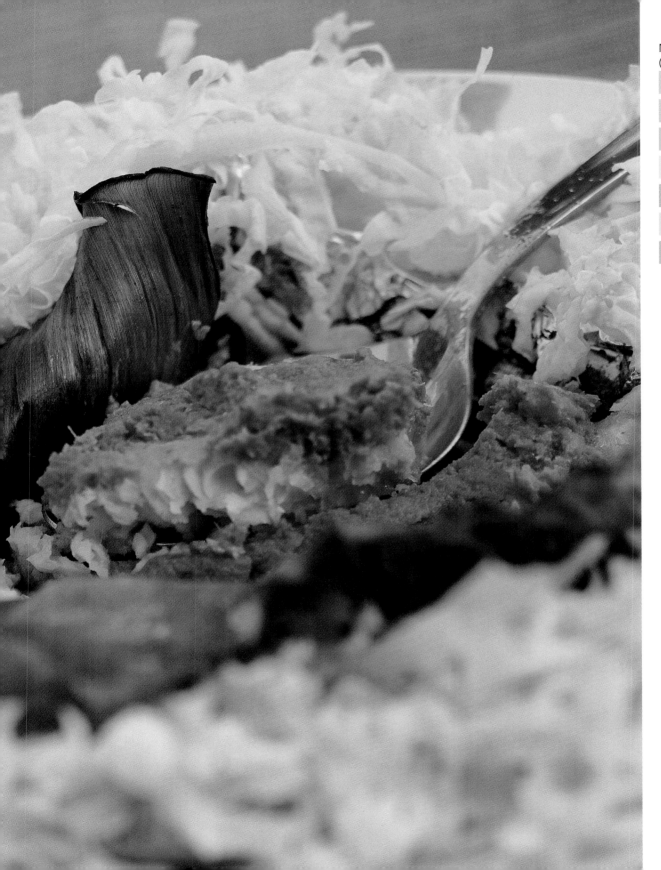

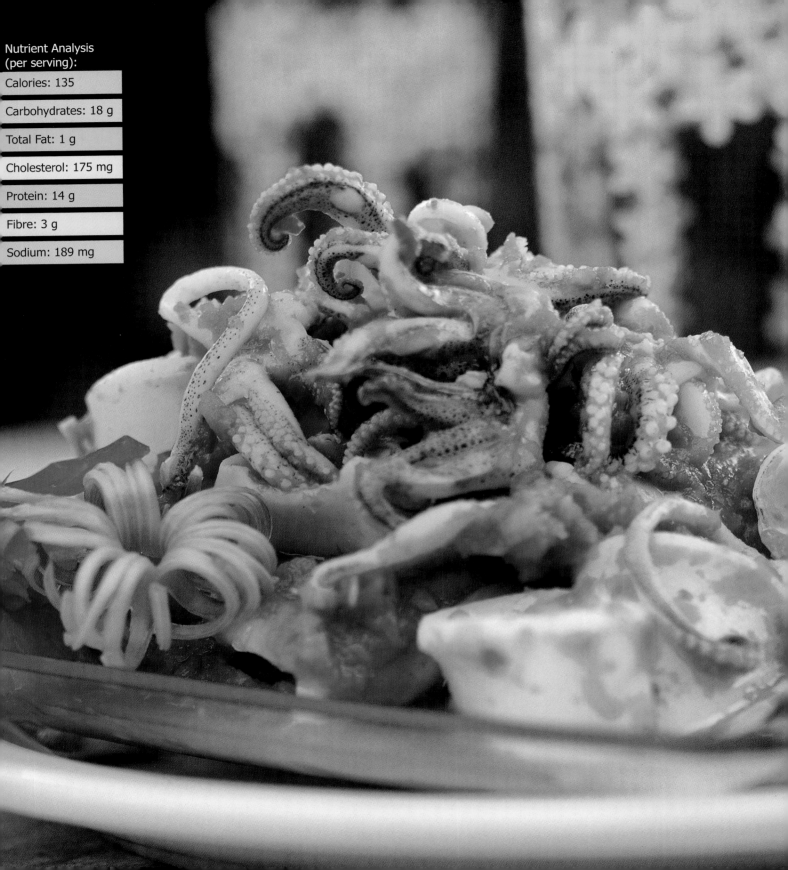

Nutrient Analysis
(per serving):

Calories: 135

Carbohydrates: 18 g

Total Fat: 1 g

Cholesterol: 175 mg

Protein: 14 g

Fibre: 3 g

Sodium: 189 mg

SOTONG SAMBAL

Nick's culinary jottings: We all love *sambal*. However, the oily kind seems to be just about everywhere you look. Try this rather fresh *sambal*, it's so fresh, it's like a salad dressing. You may replace squid with prawns or fish fillets and if you are rich enough, fresh scallops, which actually taste rather different when cooked with *sambal*.

Preparation time : 20 minutes
Cooking time : 30 minutes
Serves 4

Method

- Heat a dry pan. Lightly singe squid tubes to remove excess water. Drain and set aside.

- Spray oil onto a heated pan. Add *sambal*. Cook for a few minutes, stirring constantly. Add lime juice if used.

- Add stock and simmer for 10 minutes or until rather fragrant.

- Increase heat and allow to boil until liquid is halved. Adjust to taste with sugar and salt.

- Add squid and boil for 2 minutes more. Remove from heat and serve hot.

Method

- Blend (process) *sambal* ingredients until well combined. The colour should be a refreshing red.

Note: *Sambal* refers to a thick chilli sauce that is fundamental to Malay cuisine.

Ingredients

Squid tubes	300 g, sliced
Spray oil	3 squirts
*Sambal**	1 recipe
Lime juice (optional)	to taste
Stock	500 ml
Sugar	1 pinch
Salt	to taste

Sambal

Red chillies	8–10
Bird's eye chillies (*cili padi*)	3 or more to taste
Tomatoes	2, peeled
Minced garlic	1 tsp
Onion	1, medium, peeled and minced
Lemon grass (*serai*)	2 stalks, thinly sliced

OTAK-OTAK

Nick's culinary jottings: You know, when I was young, I hated *otak-otak*. I thought it was gross. I guess I must have eaten a horrible *otak-otak* and then decided never to venture there again for fear of feeling sick once more. Today, *otak-otak* has since re-emerged as rather nouveau cuisine and I have had the opportunity to taste the various types and come what may, some were just divine. This is my personal recipe, which I usually teach during my classes. No coconut milk is used. Sprinkle on a little lemon juice if you wish before serving.

Preparation time : 20 minutes
Cooking time : 15 minutes
Serves 5

Ingredients

Banana leaves	
Onion	1, large, peeled
Garlic	2 cloves, peeled
Candlenuts (*buah keras*)	5
Fresh turmeric (*kunyit*)	1-cm knob, peeled
Lemon grass (*serai*)	2 stalks
Red chillies	3 or more to taste; use some bird's eye chillies (*cili padi*) for added spiciness
Dried prawn (shrimp) paste (*belacan*)	2 Tbsp
Rice milk	125 ml
Soy milk	125 ml
Kaffir lime leaves	5, finely sliced
Turmeric (*kunyit*) leaves	2, finely sliced
Eggs	2
Sugar	2 Tbsp
Salt	to taste
Mackerel	500 g, cut into bite-size pieces

Method

- Cut banana leaves into 25-cm squares. Scald and wipe dry before use.
- Grind (process) onion, garlic, candlenuts, turmeric, lemon grass, chillies and dried prawn paste to a paste.
- Transfer paste to a large bowl. Mix in rice and soy milk. Except fish, add all remaining ingredients and mix well.
- Preheat oven to 200°C (400°F).
- On each banana leaf square, spread on some mixture, add several fish pieces, then add more mixture on top to cover. Wrap as shown.
- Place parcels on a baking tray. Bake or grill for about 15 minutes, depending on size of parcels. Alternatively, steam parcels for about the same duration.

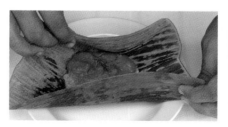
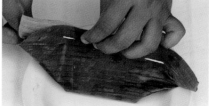
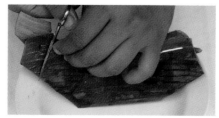

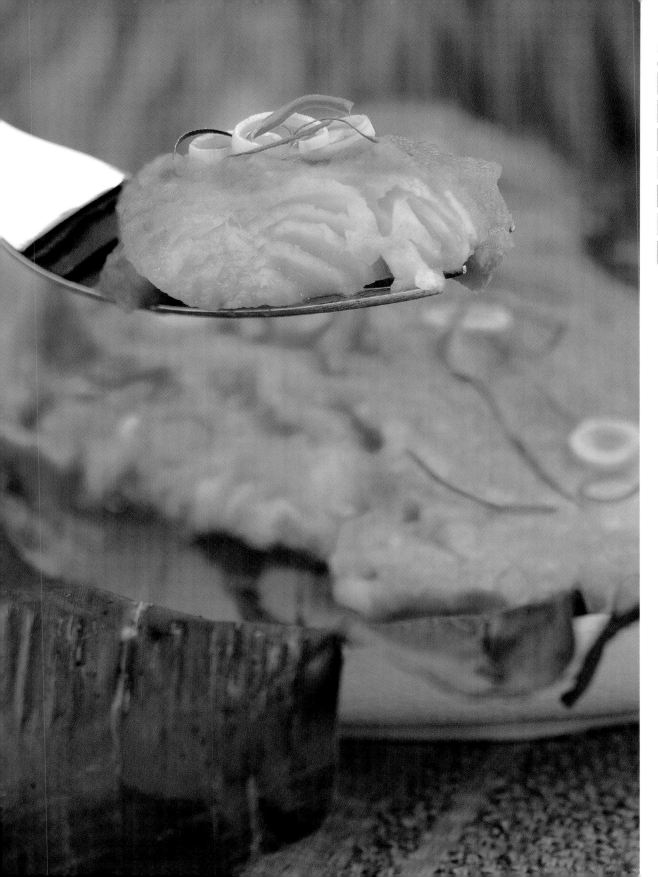

Nutrient Analysis
(per serving):

Calories: 250

Carbohydrates: 18 g

Total Fat: 9 g

Cholesterol: 159 mg

Protein: 26 g

Fibre: 1 g

Sodium: 323 mg

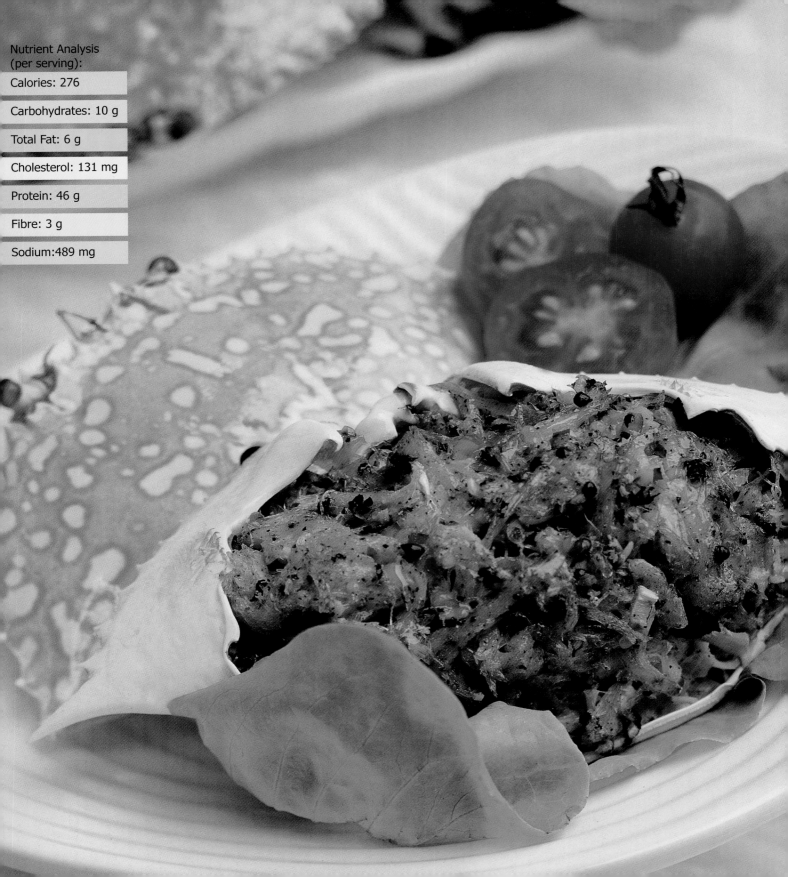

Nutrient Analysis
(per serving):

Calories: 276

Carbohydrates: 10 g

Total Fat: 6 g

Cholesterol: 131 mg

Protein: 46 g

Fibre: 3 g

Sodium:489 mg

BAKED CRAB WITH SHARK'S FIN

Nick's culinary jottings: Now, I am not a fan of crab unless mum is next to me to pull it apart and extract all the flesh for me. If I have to do it myself, I just take off what I can with my fork and leave the rest to friends and family who have no qualms about getting their fingers into the dish. Here, mud crabs, the kind with black shells that turn red when cooked, or flower crabs can be used.

Preparation time : 30 minutes
Cooking time : 20 minutes
Serves 5

Method

- Extract as much crabmeat as you can without breaking top shell.

- Combine shark's fin and stock in a pot. Simmer for a few minutes. Drain shark's fin and reserve liquid. Set both aside.

- Mash crabmeat. Add all remaining ingredients. Mix well.

- Preheat oven to 180°C (350°F).

- Combine crabmeat mixture with shark's fin. Mix in liquid 1 Tbsp at a time until mixture is pliable.

- Stuff crab shells with mixture.

- Bake crabs for 15–20 minutes, depending on size. Alternatively, steam.

Ingredients

Mud or flower crabs	2, large
Shark's fin	100 g
Stock	125 ml
Black pepper	2 Tbsp
Garlic	2 cloves, peeled and minced
Lemon grass (*serai*)	1 stalk, minced
Onion	1, small, peeled and minced
Red chillies	1 or more to taste, seeded and minced
Mustard seeds	2 Tbsp, pounded to a paste
Sugar	$^1/_2$ tsp
Egg	1
Salt	to taste

NGABAUNGDOK

Nick's culinary jottings: Originating from Myanmar, *nga baung dok* literally means "fish wrapped in banana leaves". While this may sound suspiciously like *otak-otak*, the two are not similar in any way. The ingredients and flavours are very different and this dish incorporates more vegetables than *otak-otak*, and it is always steamed. I use sole fillets simply because it is practically boneless and does not smell too fishy. Do use other kinds of fish if you like, but get those with fewer bones as it is easier and not as messy to eat.

Preparation time : 30 minutes
Cooking time : 10–15 minutes
Serves 5

Ingredients

Sole fillets	500 g, cut into bite-size pieces
Black pepper	1 Tbsp
Sesame seed oil	2 tsp
Soy milk	125 ml
Uncooked rice	2 Tbsp, freshly pounded
Coriander (cilantro)	60 g, roughly chopped
Sugar	1 pinch
Salt	to taste
Chinese cabbage leaves	6, spines removed
Banana leaves or tin foil	

Marinade

Garlic	3–4 cloves, peeled
Green chillies	3 or more to taste
Ginger	50 g, peeled
Onion	½, large, peeled
Fresh turmeric (*kunyit*)	1-cm knob, peeled

Method

- Blend (process) marinade ingredients together. Marinate fish for about 10–15 minutes.

- Except cabbage and banana leaves, combine fish and all remaining ingredients together. Mix well.

- Cut banana leaves into 25-cm squares. Scald lightly and dry before use. Use back of leaves. If unavailable, use tin foil instead.

- Wrap fish mixture as shown using cabbage leaves, then wrap over with tin foil or banana leaves.

- Steam parcels over boiling water for about 10 minutes, depending on size of parcel.

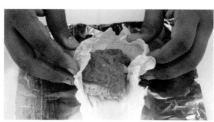 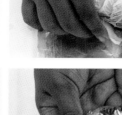
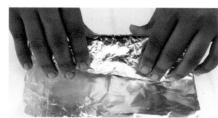 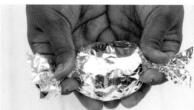

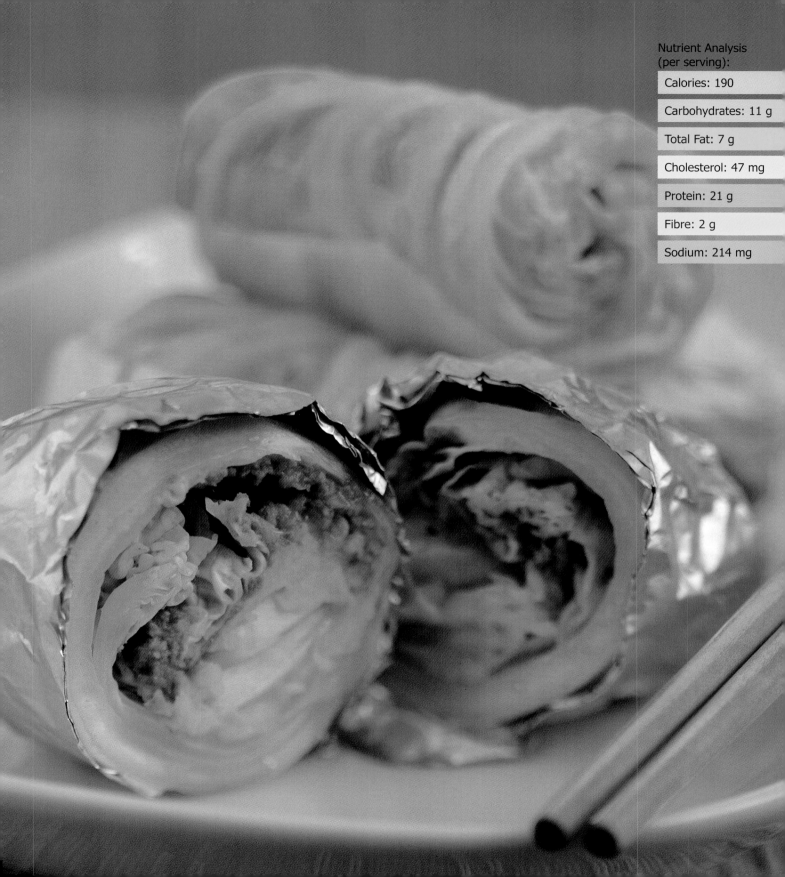

Nutrient Analysis
(per serving):

Calories: 190

Carbohydrates: 11 g

Total Fat: 7 g

Cholesterol: 47 mg

Protein: 21 g

Fibre: 2 g

Sodium: 214 mg

Nutrient Analysis
(per serving):

Calories: 205

Carbohydrates: 18 g

Total Fat: 3 g

Cholesterol: 46 mg

Protein: 29 g

Fibre: 4 g

Sodium: 259 mg

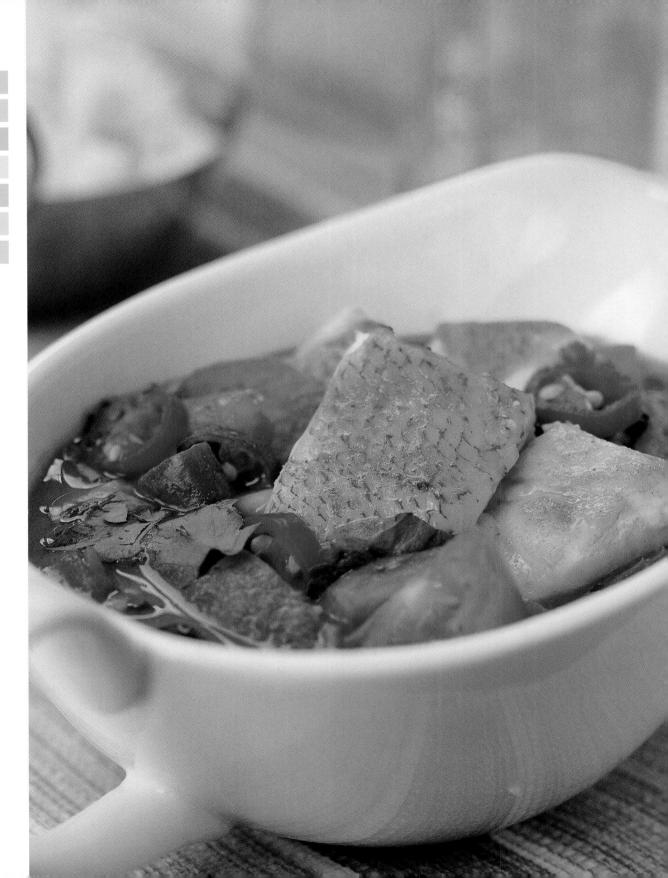

MAKER TAUKARI

Nick's culinary jottings: The Bangladeshi boys living up the road from me used to make this simple, aromatic curry that is distinctly different from what we are used to. It is very easy to make and contains no coconut cream whatsoever. The original recipe does contain a lot of oil, however. In poorer countries, oil is used to keep foods fresh as the layer of oil would protect the food throughout the day.

Preparation time : 15 minutes
Cooking time   : 30–40 minutes
Serves 4

Method

- In a dry nonstick pan over low heat, sear fish until sealed all over. When done, remove fish. Some liquid will remain in pan.

- Add stock and leave to boil. Add garlic, onion and chillies. Leave to boil for about 20 minutes.

- Add cumin, curry and chilli powders and salt to taste.

- When liquid is halved, add fish and boil for 2–3 minutes.

- Add tomatoes and coriander. Cook for about 3–5 minutes more.

Ingredients

Red snapper	500 g, cut into steak-sized pieces
Stock	500 ml
Garlic	3 cloves, peeled and coarsely chopped
Onion	1, large, peeled and coarsely chopped
Green chillies	4–5, coarsely chopped
Red chillies	2, coarsely chopped
Ground cumin	1 tsp
Fish curry powder	1 Tbsp
Chilli powder (optional)	1 Tbsp
Salt	to taste
Tomatoes	4, large, roughly chopped
Coriander (cilantro) leaves	60 g, roughly chopped

YELLOW FISH CURRY

Nick's culinary jottings: This Sri Lankan curry is mild and does not use any spice to give it flavour. Coconut milk is a big feature in most Sri Lankan curries but in our healthy case, we'll compensate by going overboard with soy milk.

Preparation time : 20 minutes
Cooking time : 35 minutes
Serves 4

Ingredients

Mackerel fillets	500 g, cut into bite-size pieces
Pepper	to taste
Onion	1, large, peeled
Garlic	4 cloves, peeled
Mustard seeds	1½ Tbsp
Ginger	30 g, peeled
Turmeric (*kunyit*)	20 g, peeled
Stock	200 ml
Curry leaves	a few sprigs; replaceable with 3 bay leaves (*daun salam*)
Soy milk	200 ml
Green chillies	3, sliced
Tomatoes (optional)	2, large, cut into segments
Salt	to taste

Method

- Season fish with a little pepper. Set aside.
- Grind (process) onion, garlic, mustard seeds, ginger and turmeric together.
- Combine stock, curry leaves and ground ingredients in a pot. Season to taste with salt. Simmer for about 20 minutes or until fragrant.
- Add soy milk and leave to boil for 10 minutes.
- Add fish and green chillies. Boil for 5 minutes more.
- If using tomatoes, add just before removing from heat.

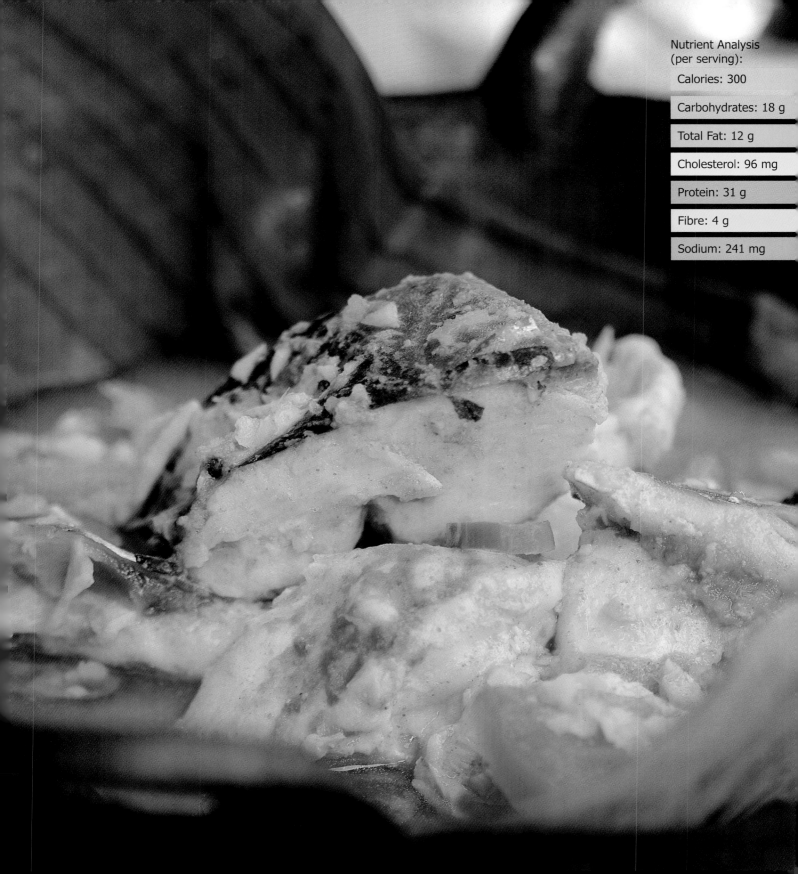

Nutrient Analysis
(per serving):

Calories: 300

Carbohydrates: 18 g

Total Fat: 12 g

Cholesterol: 96 mg

Protein: 31 g

Fibre: 4 g

Sodium: 241 mg

Nutrient Analysis
(per serving):

Calories: 275

Carbohydrates: 42 g

Total Fat: 5 g

Cholesterol: 46 mg

Protein: 17 g

Fibre: 6 g

Sodium: 246 mg

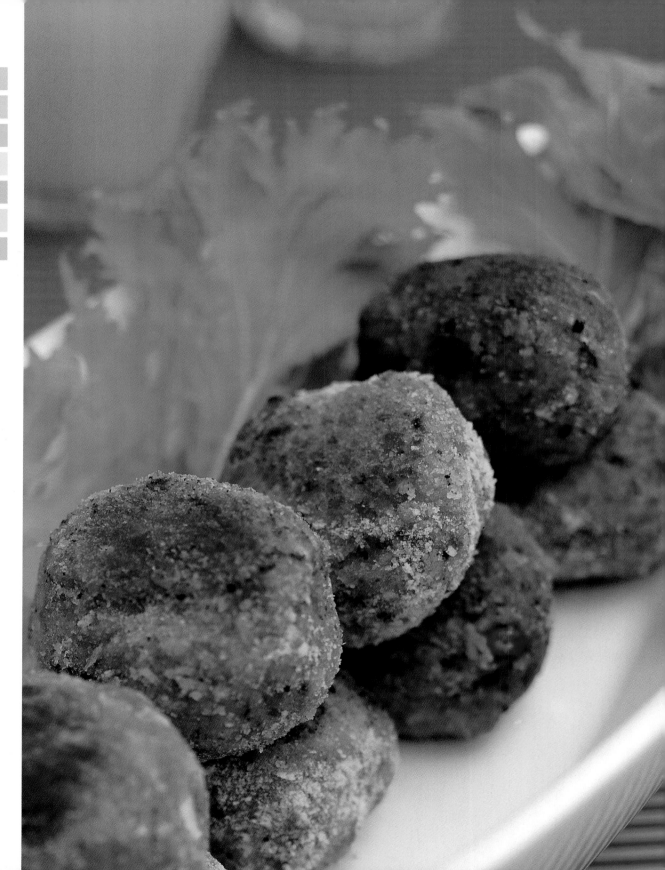

SRILANKANCUTLETS

Nick's culinary jottings: These cutlets are another Sri Lankan fish delight. Try this simple recipe, use it as part of your main meal or even as hors d'oeuvre. It is quite versatile, you know.

Preparation time : 30 minutes
Cooking time : 12–20 minutes
Serves 4

Method

- Steam fish until cooked. When done, skin and debone. Flake remaining flesh, then squeeze out excess water. Set aside.

- In a nonstick pan over low heat, sauté onion, chillies and screwpine leaves. Squeeze juices out of garlic and ginger, then add pulps to pan. Cook until fragrant. This should take about 15 minutes. Leave to cool completely.

- In a large bowl, combine flaked fish, potatoes and powdered ingredients. Add salt and pepper to taste. Stir thoroughly.

- Add sautéed ingredients. Mix well and taste. Adjust to taste with seasonings if necessary.

- Shape mixture into small rounds. When mixture is used up, coat each cutlet with egg white, then breadcrumbs.

- Heat a nonstick pan. Spray on oil. Gently place a few cutlets on pan at a time. Cook until light golden. Remember, all the ingredients are already cooked, so just get the colour and they're done.

Ingredients

Mackerel	250 g
Onion	1, peeled and minced
Chillies	2, minced
Screwpine (*pandan*) leaves	2, minced
Garlic	2 cloves, peeled and blended (processed)
Ginger	30 g, peeled and blended (processed)
Potatoes	2, large, peeled, boiled and mashed
Ground cinnamon	2 tsp
Ground cardamom	1 tsp
Ground coriander (cilantro)	1 tsp
Salt and pepper	to taste
Egg white	1, lightly beaten
Breadcrumbs	
Spray oil	2–3 squirts

Nicholas

Ahh... my favourite moment of the meal. Why don't they ever serve desserts first, follow that with the meal, and then end it with another dessert. Wouldn't that just go down well with every diner? Oops, I can see Indra shaking her head...

While most desserts can be sickeningly sweet, try to use sugar sparingly. Sugar to taste is better than the mandatory two tablespoons of sugar you know because others may not like it that sweet, or may prefer it sweeter. The desserts that I have concocted for this book range from hot to cold. They are light and also interesting to the palate, so go ahead and try them, I think you can afford that second piece too, you know.

Indra

When we say balanced diet, Nicholas' idea of having dessert upon dessert won't cut it. Sorry buddy, nice try though. Desserts are meant to be like the proverbial icing on a cake, to round off a fantastic meal as it were and hence, the portions should be politely petite. There's a reason why dessert is not served on a dinner plate. If you come face to face with a mammoth-sized dessert, be gracious and share it with the rest of your party at the table. Use the excuse that true friendships start with shared calories and fat grams if you have to!

What I love about the dessert recipes here is that they are light and full of fruits. The natural sweetness of fruit allows you to cut down on the sugar used. Some of you may choose to use artificial sweeteners to replace sugar so as to cut down on calories. There are three main types of artificial sweeteners — saccharin (Sweet 'N Low), aspartame (EQUAL or Nutrasweet) and acesulfame-K (Sweet One). Please see my notes at the end of each recipe to see which artificial sweetener is recommended for that recipe.

All nutrient analyses for *Desserts & Tea Time Treats* were calculated based on the assumption that real sugar was used.

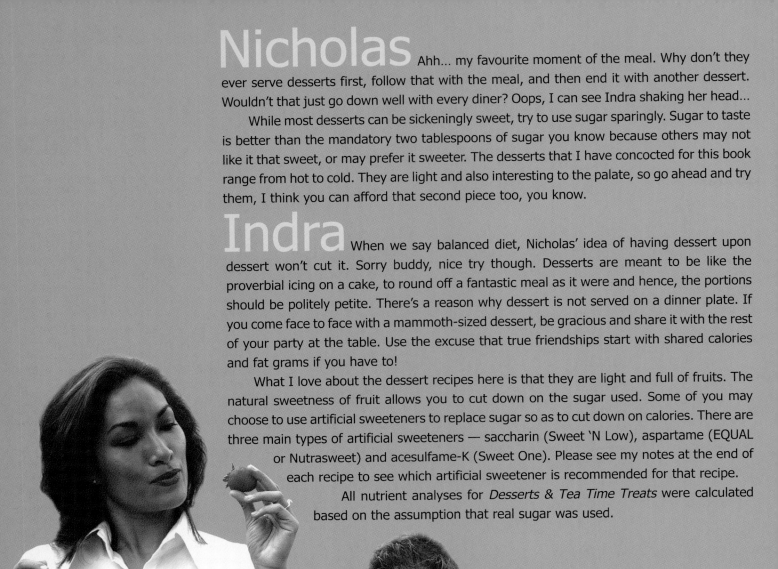

DESSERTS AND TEA TIME TREATS

FRESHFRUITSORBET

Nick's culinary jottings: This very easy to make fresh fruit sorbet is a little similar to Italian *gelato*. A truly refreshing dessert, tea time treat or snack, this sorbet, in fact, can be had any time of the day. It's absolutely fat-free too.

Preparation time : 20 minutes (does not include freezing)
Cooking time : 5 minutes
Serves 4

Ingredients

Water	250 ml
Sugar	225 g
Strawberries	200 g, frozen
Lime juice	60 ml
Extra strawberries	quantity as desired, roughly chopped
Sprigs of mint	

Method

- Combine water and sugar in a pot. Boil until sugar is dissolved. Leave to cool. Freeze cooled liquid to develop some ice. Set freezer to the coldest possible temperature.

- In a blender (processor), combine iced sugar syrup, frozen strawberries and lime juice. Blend thoroughly. Transfer to a container with a lid. Cover and freeze until almost hard.

- Return to blender and blend for about 30–40 seconds. Remove and add extra strawberries. Refreeze until done.

- Serve with a sprig of mint.

Nicholas' tip: You can replace strawberries with a host of other fruits, including mangoes, honeydew melon, rock melon (cantaloupe), plain lime and lemon (but add some lemon zest or grated rind) and even the humble green apple. In fact, just about any fleshy fruit will do as well.

Indra's note: If you like, you can use saccharin sweetener (Sweet 'N Low) instead of sugar. 225 g sugar = 12 sachets or 4 tsp saccharin. As this recipe involves cooking, aspartame sweeteners (such as EQUAL or Nutrasweet) should be avoided because they give a bitter aftertaste with heat.

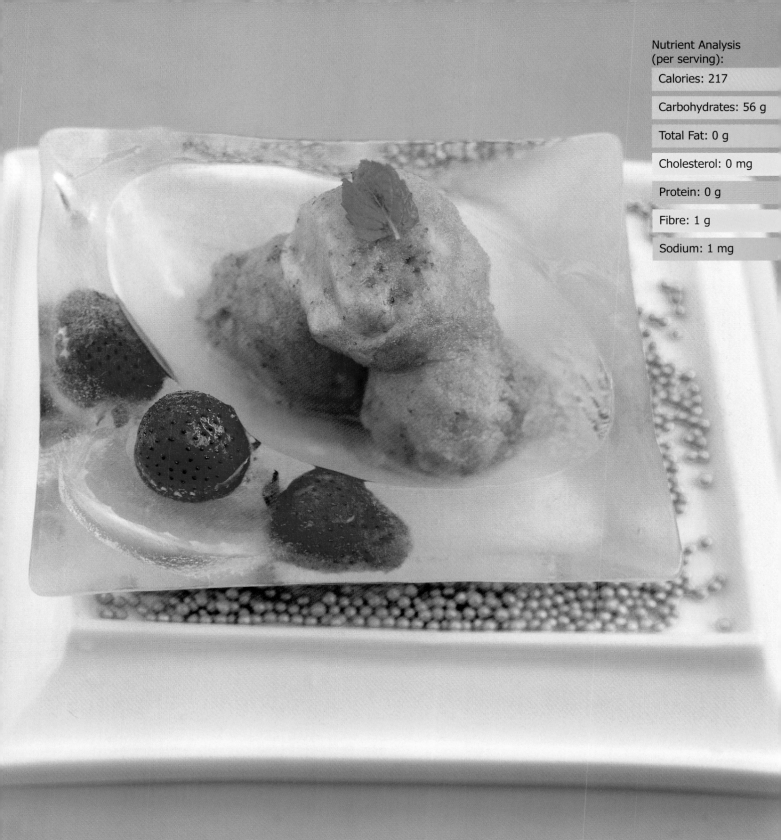

Nutrient Analysis
(per serving):

Calories: 204

Carbohydrates: 48 g

Total Fat: 1 g

Cholesterol: 0 mg

Protein: 3 g

Fibre: 5 g

Sodium: 15 mg

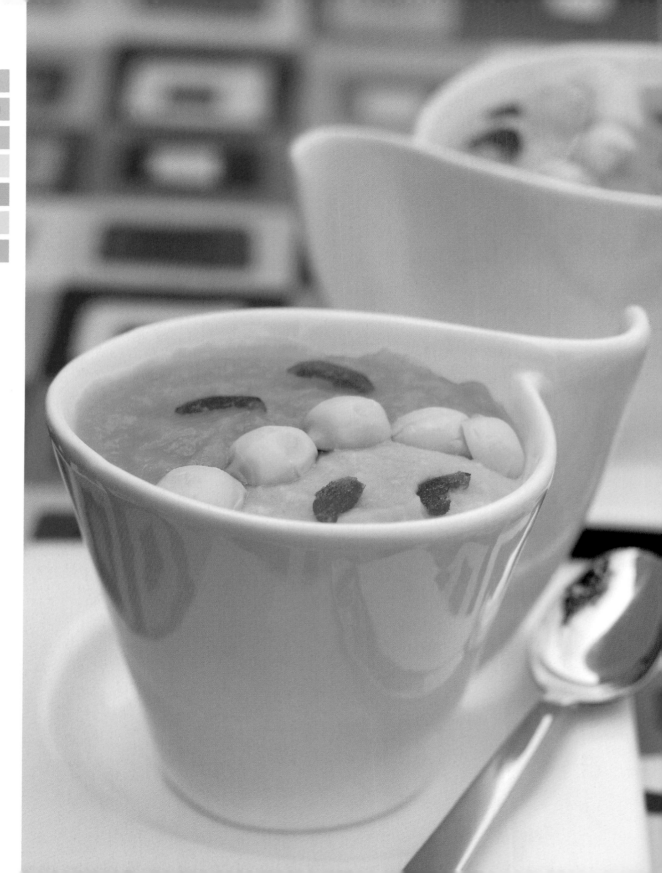

YAM PASTE WITH PUMPKIN AND LOTUS SEED

Nick's culinary jottings: This rich Taiwanese dessert should be eaten hot. It does not taste nice when it is cold as it gets lumpy.

Method

- Separately steam yam and pumpkin for 20 minutes or until soft.
- Separately mash yam and pumpkin to a paste when still hot.
- Split each lotus seed in two. Remove green bitter cores if still attached.
- Add 1 tsp sugar to pumpkin paste, mix well.
- Mix yam paste with sugar to taste, then wrap with tin foil and steam for 20 minutes.
- To serve, fill half a serving cup or bowl with pumpkin paste and the other half with yam. Arrange a few lotus seed halves on top. Decorate with thinly sliced glacé (candied) cherries if desired.

Preparation time : 30 minutes
Cooking time : 30 minutes
Serves 4

Ingredients

Yam	500 g, peeled and sliced
Pumpkin	100 g, peeled and sliced
Lotus seeds	10, boiled until just cooked, not soft; replaceable with gingko nuts
Castor (superfine) sugar or saccharin sweetener	to taste

POACHEDPEARSWITHCRYSTALLISED GINGERANDLEMONZESTINREDWINE

Preparation time : 30 minutes
Cooking time : 20 minutes
Serves 4

Nick's culinary jottings: Don't let this recipe with the long name put you off because it is easy and very eye-catching when served to your guests. It looks like it came out of some five-star restaurant!

Ingredients

Water	500 ml
Sugar or saccharin sweetener	to taste
Pears	2, peeled, halved and cored
Red wine	125 ml
Lemon zest	1 tsp and more for garnish
Crystallised ginger	2 Tbsp, cut into small pieces
Mint leaves	1 sprig

Method

- Combine water and sugar in a pot. Bring to the boil.

- Add pears. Simmer for a few minutes or until liquid is halved.

- Add wine. Simmer for a few minutes more. Adjust to taste with more sugar if needed. Add lemon zest.

- To assemble, put some crystallised ginger on a plate. Arrange pear halves upside-down looking on. Position a pair of mint leaves at the base of each half. Decorate with lemon zest.

- Serve chilled.

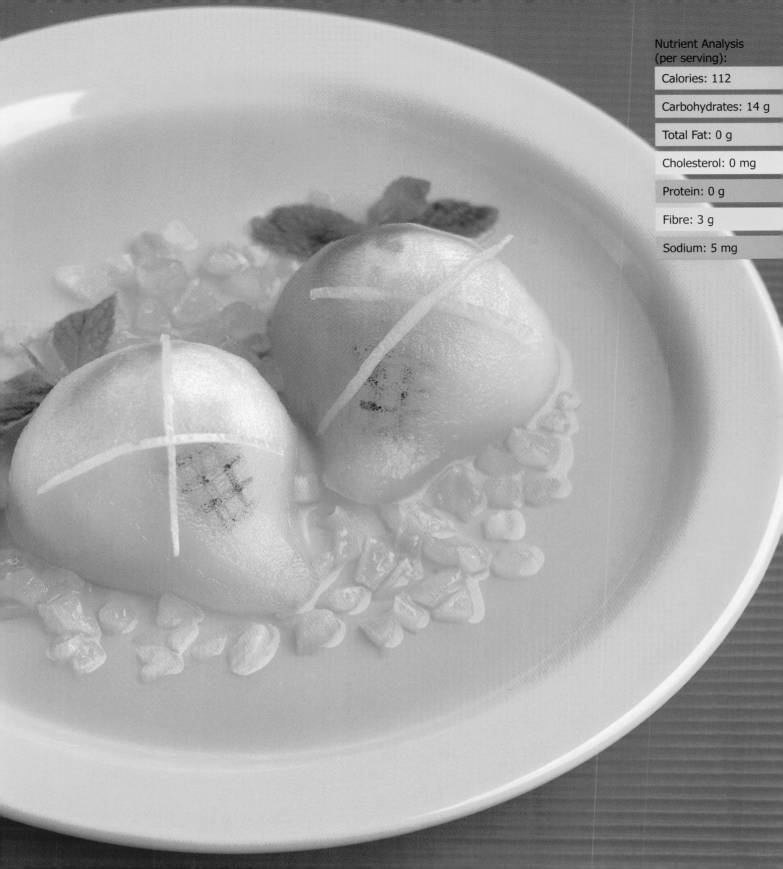

Nutrient Analysis
(per serving):

Calories: 112

Carbohydrates: 14 g

Total Fat: 0 g

Cholesterol: 0 mg

Protein: 0 g

Fibre: 3 g

Sodium: 5 mg

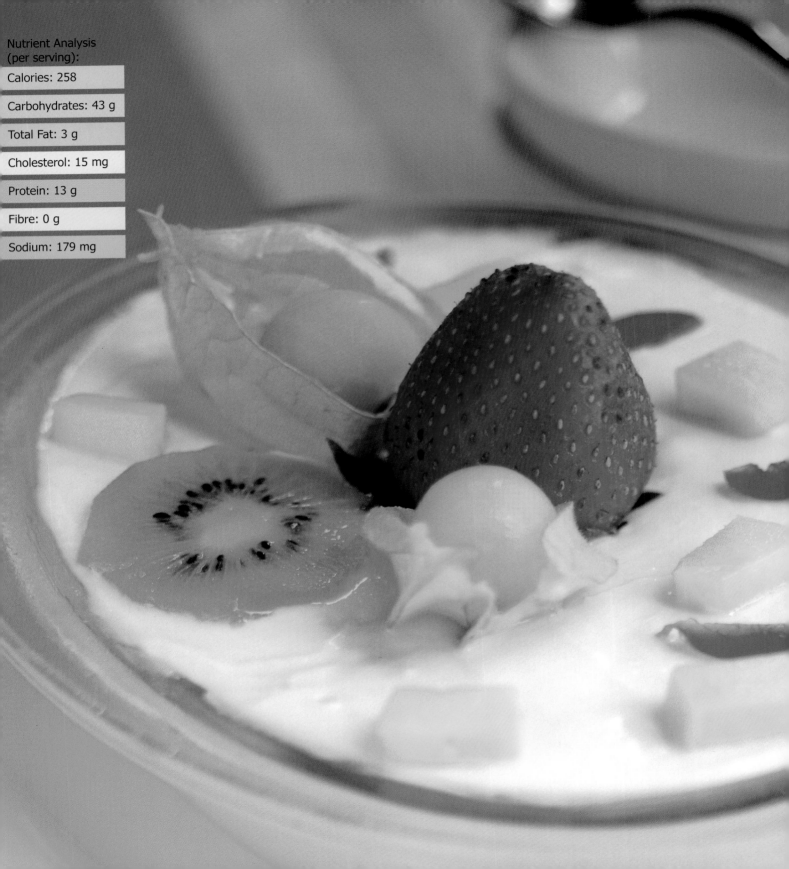

Nutrient Analysis
(per serving):

Calories: 258

Carbohydrates: 43 g

Total Fat: 3 g

Cholesterol: 15 mg

Protein: 13 g

Fibre: 0 g

Sodium: 179 mg

'CHEESECAKE' WITH FRUIT TOPPING

Nick's culinary jottings: This cheesecake recipe is almost fat-free, in that it does not have the fat content of cheesecake because it is made from yoghurt. This dessert can be made the night before and left in the refrigerator to set.

Preparation time : 180 minutes
Serves 4

Method

- Position 2 pieces of muslin cloth over a strainer with a bowl underneath and pour yoghurt onto cloth as shown.

- Tie up muslin cloth or twist it as you would a tourniquet. Put weights or something heavy on top to apply pressure. Leave to drain for a few hours.

- Squeeze from time to time. Discard water collected in bowl.

- When yoghurt is sufficiently squeezed out, it is a big lump and ready to use.

- In a mixing bowl, combine squeezed yoghurt and sugar. Use a mixer to beat until fluffy.

- Add milk and lemon juice. Continue beating until smooth and somewhat like cream cheese. Mixture should resemble thick cream.

- Transfer to a bowl or individual cups. Leave to set in refrigerator.

- Decorate with fruits of your choice.

Ingredients

Plain low-fat yoghurt	1 litre
Castor (superfine) sugar	100 g or more to taste
Low-fat milk	60 ml
Lemon juice	3 Tbsp
Fruits of your choice	

🍸 Indra's note: Since this dessert requires no cooking over heat, you can use either saccharin (Sweet 'N Low) or aspartame sweeteners (EQUAL or Nutrasweet) instead of sugar.

100 g castor sugar = 12 sachets or $3\frac{1}{2}$ tsp aspartame = 6 sachets or 2 tsp saccharin

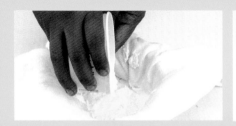 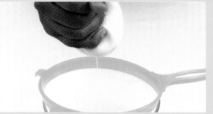

Nicholas

There is nothing like a freshly made punch or juice to pep you up any time of the day. It's rich in vitamins and depending on the fruit, can also be high in fibre. Lazy me likes a good juice in the mornings but I just don't like having to fuss with it, so sometimes, on good days, I get the housekeepers to do it for me the night before.

These days, everywhere you go, you find a myriad of juices all around. I feel that in Asia, we are luckier because we tend to add a lot of different things to juice to jazz it up. We add jellies, seeds, nuts and a whole lot of different toppings that are seldom even thought of in the West.

However, one thing different from the West though, our juices are always so overpriced. If you do a rough costing of each juice we have in this recipe you will realize how cheap it is to prepare your own. Once more, sugar is really up to you. A lot of sweetness can come from the fruit itself, you know. Choose slightly overripe fruit as the sugar content tends to be higher.

Indra

Freshly squeezed juices would probably be the next best thing for people who hate to eat fruit. A serving of fruit is equivalent to 180 ml of freshly squeezed fruit juice. When at the supermarket, be sure to read juice labels carefully. There is a large variety of juices in the market but not all of them are 100% fruit juice. Most of them are really fruit-flavoured drinks, with only a small percentage of fruit juice mixed with a large amount of sugared water. With the invention of the electric juicer, you can now easily make your own juices in a flash. Good birthday wish list addition, if you don't already own one. (Now you know what I get for MY birthdays as a dietitian!)

That said, juices as a whole cannot take the place of eating fruits whole. The simple reason being that you get tons of fibre from the whole fruit, so as part of your healthy meal plan, have both whole fruit and fruit juices.

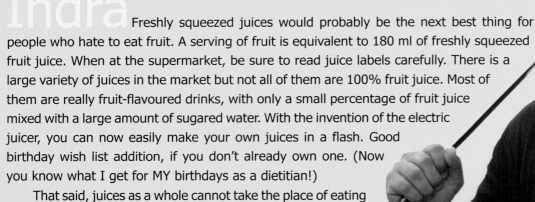

JUICES AND SMOOTHIES

HEALTHY STRAWBERRY SHAKE

Preparation time : 5 minutes
Serves 2

Nick's culinary jottings: These drinks are so cheap to make at home and yet, when you get them at coffee shops, they are exorbitant! Try the following juice concoction and you will see how simple it really is.

Ingredients

Strawberries	1 punnet (approximately 250 g)
Strawberry low-fat yogurt	1 tub (125 ml)
Skimmed or soy milk	250 ml
Wheat germ	1 Tbsp
Sugar, honey or artificial sweetener	to taste
Ice cubes	

Method

- Combine all ingredients in a blender (processor). Blend at full speed.

- Pour into a glass and serve immediately. Garnish with a strawberry.

- Top with extra ice cubes for a lighter, more refreshing drink if desired.

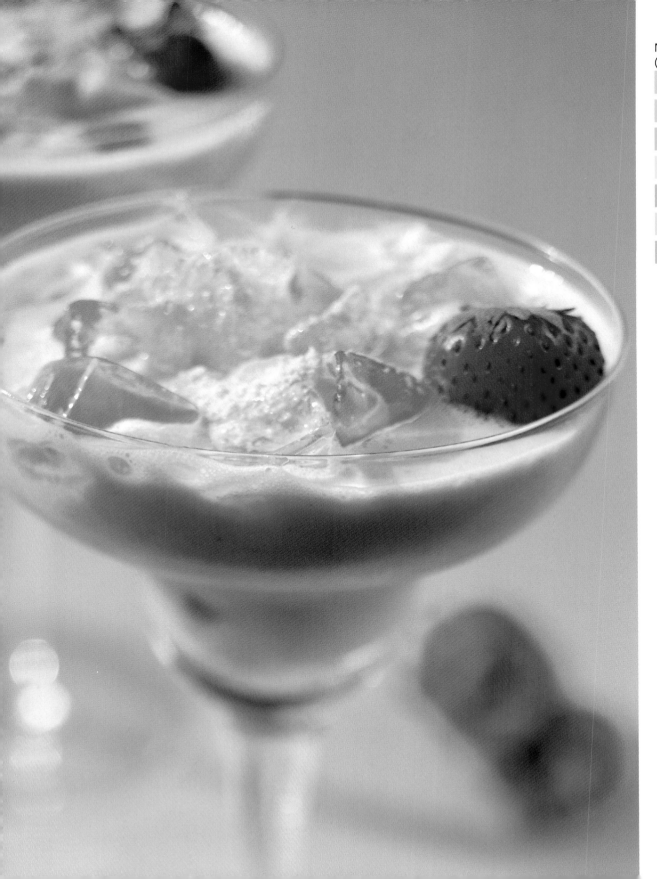

Nutrient Analysis
(per serving):

Calories: 216

Carbohydrates: 41 g

Total Fat: 2 g

Cholesterol: 13 mg

Protein: 11 g

Fibre: 4 g

Sodium: 116 mg

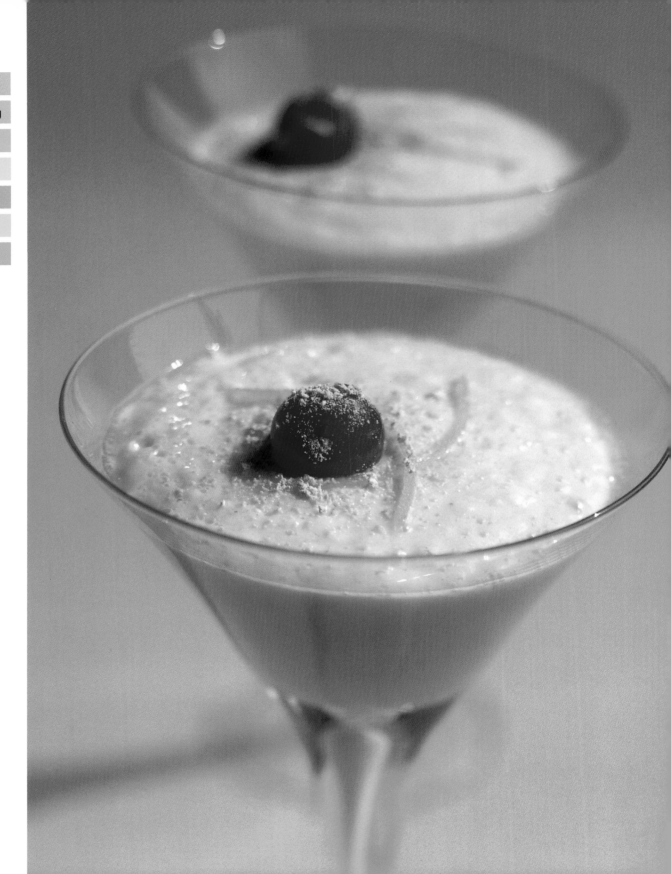

Nutrient Analysis
(per serving):

Calories: 304

Carbohydrates: 61 g

Total Fat: 4 g

Cholesterol: 16 mg

Protein: 11 g

Fibre: 8 g

Sodium: 148 mg

SOURSOP SMOOTHIE

Preparation time : 5 minutes
Serves 2

Method

- Except nutmeg and lemon peel, combine all other ingredients in a blender (processor). Blend well.

- To serve, sprinkle on a tiny bit of ground nutmeg or garnish with julienned lemon peel. Serve chilled.

Ingredients

Soursop pulp	500 g
Lime juice	3 tsp
Low-fat vanilla ice cream	1 scoop
Yoghurt	2 scoops
Sugar syrup or artificial sweetener	to taste
Ice cubes	
Ground nutmeg	
Lemon peel (optional)	

STAR FRUIT AND KIWI PICKERUPPER

Ingredients

Kiwi fruit	2, quite ripe and peeled
Star fruit	1, ripe
Lime juice	to taste
Sugar syrup or artificial sweetener	to taste
Ice cubes	

Method

- Combine all ingredients in a blender (processor). Blend at full speed.

- Pour into a tall glass and serve immediately. Garnish with slices of star fruit and kiwi.

- Top with extra ice cubes for a lighter and more refreshing drink if desired.

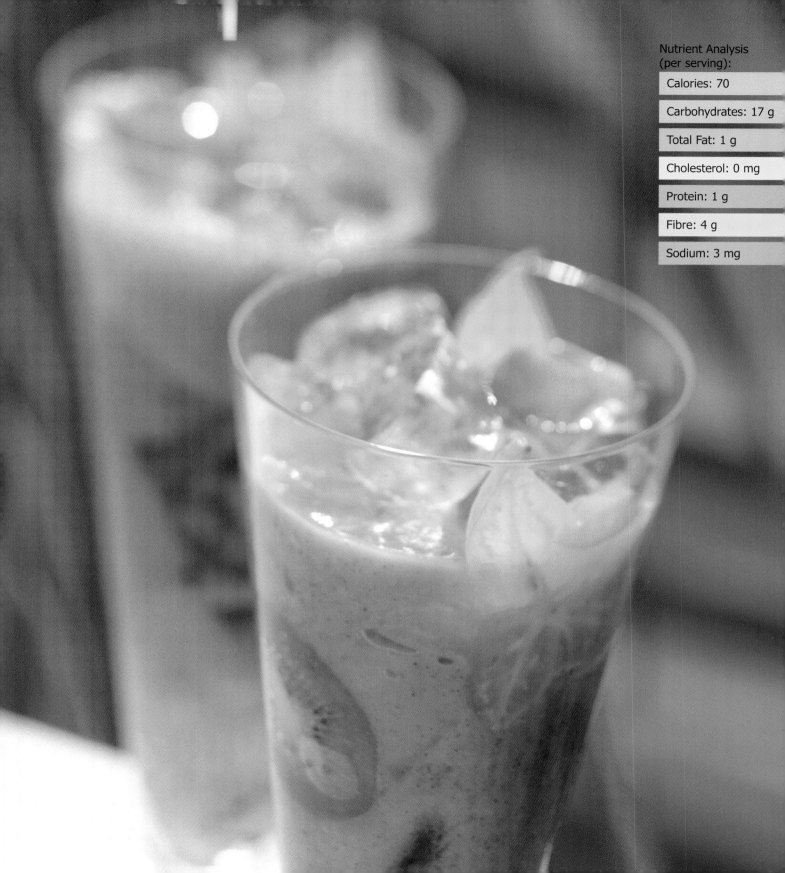

Nutrient Analysis
(per serving):

Calories: 70

Carbohydrates: 17 g

Total Fat: 1 g

Cholesterol: 0 mg

Protein: 1 g

Fibre: 4 g

Sodium: 3 mg

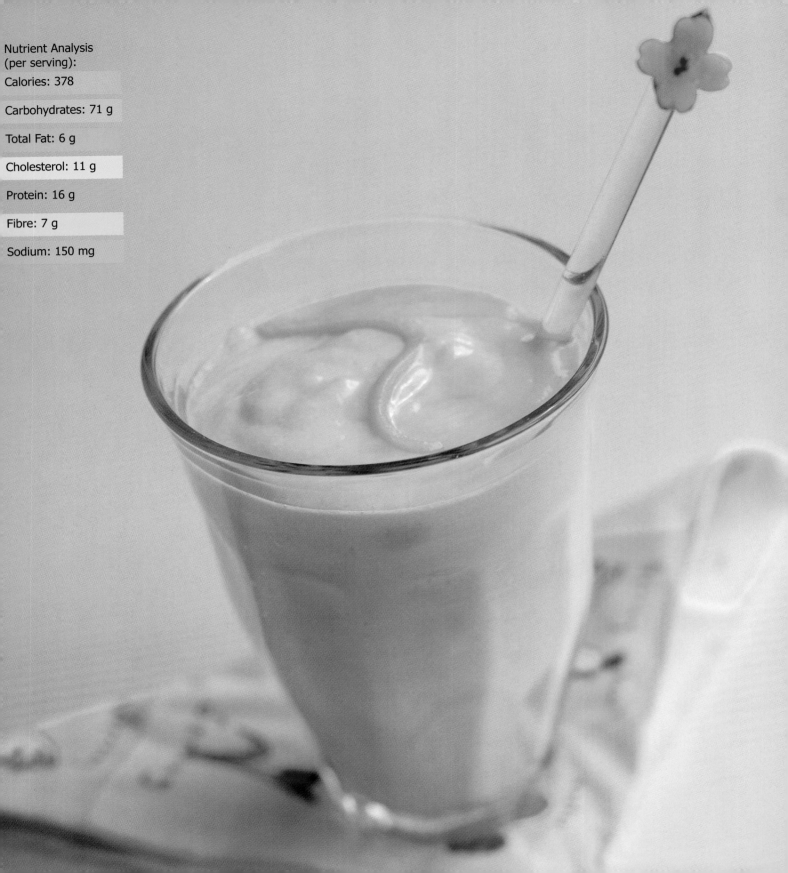

Nutrient Analysis
(per serving):

Calories: 378

Carbohydrates: 71 g

Total Fat: 6 g

Cholesterol: 11 g

Protein: 16 g

Fibre: 7 g

Sodium: 150 mg

MANGOLASSI

Nick's culinary jottings: Mango lassi has a strong following for some odd reason. It is so easy to make and when made at home, you can adjust the amount of mango to your liking.

Preparation time : 5 minutes
Serves 2

Method

- Blend (process) all ingredients until thick and creamy.
- Pour into tall glasses. Garnish as desired. Serve immediately.

Ingredients

Mango pulp	450 g or more to taste
Plain low-fat yoghurt	375 g
Soy milk	250 ml
Sugar or artificial sweetener	to taste
Ice cubes	

Garnishing

Julienned mango pulp (optional)

Crushed pistachios (optional)

Sprigs of mint (optional)

WEIGHTS AND MEASURES

Quantities for this book are given in Metric and American (spoon and cup) measures. Standard spoon and cup measurements used are: 1 teaspoon = 5 ml, 1 dessertspoon = 10 ml, 1 tablespoon = 15 ml, 1 cup = 250 ml. All measures are level unless otherwise stated.

LIQUID AND VOLUME MEASURES

Metric	Imperial	American
5 ml	1/6 fl oz	1 teaspoon
10 ml	1/3 fl oz	1 dessertspoon
15 ml	1/2 fl oz	1 tablespoon
60 ml	2 fl oz	1/4 cup (4 tablespoons)
85 ml	2 1/2 fl oz	1/3 cup
90 ml	3 fl oz	3/8 cup (6 tablespoons)
125 ml	4 fl oz	1/2 cup
180 ml	6 fl oz	3/4 cup
250 ml	8 fl oz	1 cup
300 ml	10 fl oz (1/2 pint)	1 1/4 cups
375 ml	12 fl oz	1 1/2 cups
435 ml	14 fl oz	1 3/4 cups
500 ml	16 fl oz	2 cups
625 ml	20 fl oz (1 pint)	2 1/2 cups
750 ml	24 fl oz (1 1/5 pints)	3 cups
1 litre	32 fl oz (1 3/5 pints)	4 cups
1.25 litres	40 fl oz (2 pints)	5 cups
1.5 litres	48 fl oz (2 2/5 pints)	6 cups
2.5 litres	80 fl oz (4 pints)	10 cups

DRY MEASURES

Metric	Imperial
30 grams	1 ounce
45 grams	1 1/2 ounces
55 grams	2 ounces
70 grams	2 1/2 ounces
85 grams	3 ounces
100 grams	3 1/2 ounces
110 grams	4 ounces
125 grams	4 1/2 ounces
140 grams	5 ounces
280 grams	10 ounces
450 grams	16 ounces (1 pound)
500 grams	1 pound, 1 1/2 ounces
700 grams	1 1/2 pounds
800 grams	1 3/4 pounds
1 kilogram	2 pounds, 3 ounces
1.5 kilograms	3 pounds, 4 1/2 ounces
2 kilograms	4 pounds, 6 ounces

OVEN TEMPERATURE

	°C	°F	Gas Regulo
Very slow	120	250	1
Slow	150	300	2
Moderately slow	160	325	3
Moderate	180	350	4
Moderately hot	190/200	370/400	5/6
Hot	210/220	410/440	6/7
Very hot	230	450	8
Super hot	250/290	475/550	9/10

LENGTH

Metric	Imperial
0.5 cm	1/4 inch
1 cm	1/2 inch
1.5 cm	3/4 inch
2.5 cm	1 inch

ABBREVIATION

tsp	teaspoon
dsp	dessertspoon
Tbsp	tablespoon
g	gram
ml	millilitre